miniature HORSES

miniature HORSES

A Veterinary Guide for Owners and Breeders

Rebecca L. Frankeny
VMD, MS, Diplomate ACVS

Contributing Author
Steven Duren, PhD

Illustrations
Kathi Haworth

Foreword
Ron Scheuring, DVM

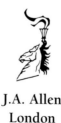

J.A. Allen
London

TABLE OF CONTENTS

To my husband Mike,
for his love, support, enthusiasm,
and patience

ACKNOWLEDGMENTS

MY FIRST WORDS of thanks go to my client and Miniature horse owner, Kim Sweatt. In response to her frustration at the lack of basic veterinary information on Miniature horses, I commented, "Someone needs to write a book." Her reply, "Maybe you should write a book," was what set this whole project in motion.

I would also like to express my immense appreciation to Michelle and Monty Meacham and Laura Meacham for their unrelenting enthusiasm and encouragement for this book and for sharing their experience and expertise as I gathered information. For entrusting me with the care of their lovely animals, I am grateful to all my Miniature horse clients on a daily basis.

I am forever indebted to my group of proofreaders and "at-home editors" who spent endless hours reviewing my manuscript: my forever patient husband Mike, my friends and neighbors Sue and Cal Reed, and my dear friend and confidant, Dr. Nancy Diehl. Thanks also to Dr. Ron Scheuring, Dr. Steve Duren, Dr. Joanne Kramer, Dr. Sue McDonnell, Dr. Tim Evans, and Kitty and Bill Pearce for their suggestions and contributions to the manuscript.

Finally, this book would never have happened were it not for the artistic talent of my great friend and illustrator, Kathi Haworth. Somehow, she managed to find time in between a husband, two small children, riding instructions, and training horses to create the illustrations that clarify the text of the manuscript. Sharing this project with her has made it even more special to me.

IT IS WITH personal and professional respect that I take this opportunity to introduce *Miniature Horses: A Veterinary Guide for Owners and Breeders.*

For the past twenty-two years, I have enjoyed the unique experience of not only breeding, showing, and training the Miniature horse, but serving the industry through administration via directorship as well as chairing and participating on many committees. As a Doctor of Veterinary Medicine in the early years of this breed, I noticed that several subtle differences in these small horses began to emerge. At that time, there were not enough breeders, owners, or Miniature horses to make it worthwhile for research time and money to be spent on the breed, and it was questionable as to whether people's passion for, and talents of these horses would be embraced and noticed by other horse enthusiasts. Through the combined efforts of some determined and dedicated individuals, and the intense heart of those "foundation horses," we are now enjoying these exciting newcomers in the equine industry.

Today, the Miniature horse industry looks at well over one hundred thousand registered horses, with breeders in abundance not only throughout the Americas but also throughout the world. The American Miniature horse enjoys a flourishing show circuit. The marketing efforts of the American Miniature Horse Association, American Miniature Horse Registry, as well as private farms provide the public with an abundance of information spawning interest and creating business and hobby opportunities.

Early on, when my colleagues and other equine professionals had little or no information, I would find myself professionally challenged and continually on a quest for any resources that would satisfy my professional appetite for the ongoing and critical care of the Miniature horse. I have foaled out over four hundred Miniature horse mares, and performed and assisted in dystocia and C-section deliveries as well as colic and other medical procedures pertaining specifically to the Miniature horse. *Miniature Horses* would have been an invaluable asset to not only myself, but to clients and friends both personally and professionally.

It is within these pages of *Miniature Horses* that Dr. Rebecca Frankeny has compiled, with brilliant accuracy and clarity, this long overdue reference book. She has taken the hours of her daily experience, nights of countless emergencies and critical-care decisions with the Miniature horse and her clients, and compiled a reference piece that will be a "must have" on the book shelf of not only every Miniature horse owner but veterinarians as well. (Forget the bookshelf. Put it in the barn!)

This well thought-out and well illustrated book contains valuable information essential to the breed. It provides the readers a better perspective on their horses and extends their knowledge by assisting them to ask educated questions.

Dr. Frankeny's information is derived from not only her professional integrity to this breed and her dedication to the veterinary profession, but her dedication to the horses entrusted to her care. In my opinion, the entire Miniature horse industry will be enriched and enlightened by her work. It is my pleasure to be able to thank her for giving so generously of her time and talent to recognize the Miniature horse in this very special way. Her work is indeed long overdue and indeed a requirement for serious Miniature horse enthusiasts.

Such a gift to the Miniature horse breed!

Ron Scheuring, DVM
Sami's Lil Horse Ranch

A GLOSSARY OF unusual words and veterinary terms is on page 153. The first time each of these words is mentioned in the text, you will see it in bold-faced type. This is to alert you to the fact that there is a detailed explanation of the word at the end of the book.

The Unique Medical Concerns
of the Miniature Horse

THROUGH YEARS OF selective breeding, Miniature horses have developed into true scaled-down versions of full-sized horses. However, despite the similarity in appearance to their large distant relatives, with respect to veterinary care, Miniature horses cannot be viewed simply as smaller versions of full-sized horses. The rate of occurrence, diagnosis, and treatment of many diseases are affected by their small size and unique physiological and metabolic demands.

There are many excellent books and magazines on equine health care for owners of full-sized horses. Unfortunately, the information available in these publications is not always applicable to Miniature horse owners. For example, abnormalities such as navicular disease, osteochondrosis (OCD), and laryngeal hemiplegia (roaring) that are widespread in the large horse population are rarely, if ever, seen in Miniature horses. On the other hand, hepatic lipidosis, a form of liver failure that can occur during times of food deprivation, is very rare in full-sized horses, but quite common in Miniatures.

The purpose of writing this book is to educate readers on the health issues that are of special concern or present unique challenges in diagnosis or treatment in Miniature horses. By limiting the subject matter to Miniature horses, the text presents each problem in more detail than is normally covered in books on equine health care. The rationale behind the greater detail is that the added information will help owners in the prevention and early recognition of common medical problems and prepare them for what they may expect if their horse becomes ill.

This book is not meant to be a "how to be your own veterinarian" manual. There is no substitute for the care and guidance provided by an experienced veterinarian. However, a veterinarian's most important partner is a knowledgeable, observant horse owner. It is my hope that the information provided in this book will help strengthen the partnership between the Miniature horse owner and the veterinarian, and lead to longer, healthier lives for these entertaining and endearing animals.

CHAPTER 1

The Musculoskeletal System

THE MUSCULOSKELETAL SYSTEM is made up of the bones, joints, muscles, **tendons,** and **ligaments** that provide the means for locomotion to the horse and protect the vital organs of the body.

There are many important differences between full-sized horses and Miniature horses with respect to the musculoskeletal system. In general, Miniature horses experience far fewer musculoskeletal problems than large horses. Lamenesses such as navicular disease and arthritis, which are very common in full-sized horses, are rarely seen in Miniatures. This is probably due to their small size and the fact that they are rarely required to carry additional weight. On the other hand, some abnormalities such as persistent soft-tissue **laxity** and patellar **luxation** in foals are more common in Miniature horses than in full-sized animals. Because they reach their growth potential at a younger age than full-sized foals, growth abnormalities must be resolved at an earlier age in Miniature horses. Injuries such as fractures and patellar luxations that carry a guarded prognosis in large horses can often be successfully repaired in Miniature horses.

After a general review of anatomic terms and a detailed description of the structure, function, and care of the hoof, this chapter addresses those diseases and injuries of the musculoskeletal system that are common or present unique concerns with respect to treatment in Miniature horses: hoof diseases, abnormalities of growth, stifle abnormalities, and fractures. Possible causes of the abnormality, how a diagnosis is reached, treatment options, and prognosis will be discussed where applicable. The goal is to provide owners with information that will help them prevent common lamenesses, recognize the early signs of a problem, and prepare them for how their veterinarian may treat the abnormality.

Basic Anatomy of the Horse

Understanding basic anatomical terms is essential to any discussion on the musculoskeletal system, and it is beneficial when communicating

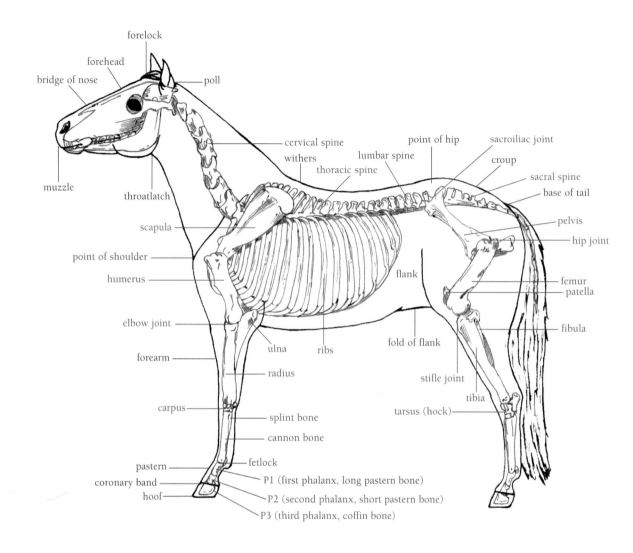

forelock
forehead
bridge of nose
poll
cervical spine
withers
lumbar spine
thoracic spine
point of hip
sacroiliac joint
croup
sacral spine
base of tail
muzzle
throatlatch
scapula
pelvis
hip joint
point of shoulder
humerus
flank
femur
patella
elbow joint
ulna
ribs
fibula
forearm
fold of flank
radius
stifle joint
tibia
carpus
tarsus (hock)
splint bone
cannon bone
pastern
fetlock
coronary band
P1 (first phalanx, long pastern bone)
hoof
P2 (second phalanx, short pastern bone)
P3 (third phalanx, coffin bone)

1. Common names of equine
anatomic structures. Skeletal parts
are labeled in blue, and body parts
in green.

with veterinarians and other horse owners. Figure 1.1 provides the common names of equine anatomic structures.

Other anatomic terms that are essential for precise communication in veterinary medicine are descriptors of position and direction that are used to define relative positions on the body. The terms that will be most commonly used in this chapter are **medial** and **lateral.** Medial structures are those that lie toward the middle of the horse and lateral structures lie toward the outside of the horse (fig. 1.2). For instance, the medial side of the leg is the inside half of the leg, and the lateral side of the leg is the outside half.

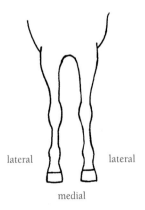

1.2 The terms "medial" and "lateral" are used to describe structures that lie toward the middle and the outside of the horse respectively.

The Hoof and its Associated Structures

The equine foot is a masterpiece of engineering. Not only is the hoof wall tough enough to protect the bone and sensitive tissues within the hoof, but it also dissipates the concussive forces that occur each time the hoof strikes the ground, forces that can exceed the weight of the horse by several fold during normal movement. In addition, the expansion and contraction of the elastic, shock-absorbing structures of the hoof and soft tissues within, act to stimulate the blood flow that nourishes the foot. Knowing the structure and function of the foot is an important step to understanding proper routine care of the hoof and the common lameness problems seen in this part of the leg.

The Anatomy of the Foot

Skeleton
The main bone in the foot is the third phalanx or coffin bone (fig. 1.3a). It sits within the hoof and its shape is very similar to the external shape of the hoof wall. The coffin bone and the second phalanx, also known as the short pastern bone, form the coffin joint (fig. 1.3b). Only about half of the second phalanx is within the hoof wall.

Directly behind the coffin bone, adjacent to the coffin joint, is a small, boat-shaped bone called the navicular bone (fig. 1.3c and k). This bone acts as a pivot point for the deep digital flexor tendon as it makes a bend toward its attachment on the ground surface of the coffin bone. There is a small, fluid-filled envelope called the navicular that lies between the navicular bone and the deep digital flexor tendon (fig. 1.3d). It provides a lubricated surface for the sliding of the flexor tendon over the bone.

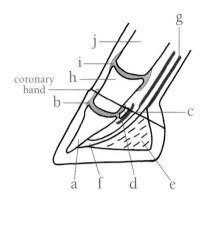

a: coffin bone (third phalanx)
b: coffin joint
c: navicular bone
d: navicular bursa
e: digital cushion
f: deep digital flexor tendon
g: tendon sheath
h: second phalanx (short pastern bone)
i: pastern joint
j: first phalanx (long pastern bone)
k: view of navicular bone from the front

1.3 The structures of the foot. This diagram shows a cross-section view of the inside of the hoof.

Hoof Wall

The structures of the foot are enclosed within the hoof wall. Because the hoof wall is the main weight-bearing structure of the foot, a healthy wall is a necessary prerequisite for a sound horse.

The wall is a tough, protective box made of keratinized epithelium, similar to our fingernails. It is produced by the coronary band (fig. 1.3) and it takes nine to twelve months for a new wall to completely grow out. The rate of growth is dependent on the environment, with the slowest rate of growth occurring under cold, dry conditions. Other factors that can adversely affect the rate of growth and health of the hoof wall are decreased exercise, injury to the coronary band, illness, and nutritional deficiencies.

The hoof wall is coupled to the coffin bone by an interconnection of sensitive and insensitive finger-like projections of tissue called *laminae* (fig. 1.4). The effect is a microscopic tongue-in-groove design. In effect, the coffin bone is suspended from the hoof wall, so that it can be said, "horses hang from their hoof walls." This demonstrates the importance of healthy laminae to a healthy foot.

Sole

The ground surface of the hoof is the sole (fig. 1.4). The function of the sole is to protect the sensitive structures of the interior of the foot. The sole grows at approximately the same rate as the wall, but unlike the wall, the sole will slough. As a result, the sole is thinner than the wall. Therefore, in an ideal foot, the sole is concave so that it does not bear weight except near its junction with the wall. It is here that the sole is thickest.

Frog

The frog sits behind the sole and is a wedge-shaped mass of keratinized epithelium (figure 1.4). It has a sponge-like consistency that is important for its shock-absorbing capacity. Like the sole, the frog will slough its outer layers if these layers are not removed by natural wear or trimming. Clefts called *sulci* lie on either side and down the center of the frog.

Collateral Cartilages

Two collateral cartilages, one medial and one lateral, are present in the hoof (fig. 1.5). The cartilages begin about the mid hoof area and extend to the heels. They extend from under the skin just above the coronary band to under the hoof wall. There is an extensive vascular network running through the collateral cartilages. The cartilages and associated vasculature are an important part of the shock-absorbing mechanism of the foot.

Digital Cushion

Directly beneath the frog, in between the collateral cartilages, lies the highly elastic digital cushion (fig. 1.3e). The cushion extends from the heel bulbs to the sole surface of the coffin bone. It attaches to the deep digital flexor tendon as the tendon inserts upon the coffin bone.

Deep Digital Flexor Tendon

The deep digital flexor tendon is not strictly a hoof structure (fig. 1.3f). The tendon originates above the **carpus** (informally called the knee[1]) or hock and terminates on the coffin bone. It is responsible for flexion of the lower two thirds of the leg. A fluid-filled envelope called a sheath surrounds the tendon starting just above the fetlock and ending just above the hoof. The tendon is of special importance when discussing the hoof because of its effect on the position of the coffin bone in a diseased foot, and because of its potential involvement in injuries to the hoof.

Blood Supply

The principle blood supply to the hoof is from the digital arteries that run down the medial and lateral side of the back of the leg. At the hoof, the arteries branch to supply the coronary band, collateral cartilages, coffin bone, and navicular bone. A large portion of the blood supply is also distributed to the sensitive tissues of the frog, sole, and wall, including the laminae. The extensive vascular networks at the coronary band and collateral cartilages act to help distribute the concussive forces acting on the hoof.

The Function of the Foot

Shock Absorbing and Circulatory Mechanisms of the Hoof

The hoof wall, sole, frog, digital cushion, collateral cartilages, and vascular network all act to decrease the force of concussion. When the foot strikes the ground, the hoof wall and the sole expand slightly. The frog contacts the ground and the force of impact is transferred to the heels of the foot and the digital cushion. This force results in an outward expansion of the digital cushion, which dissipates some of the force of concussion. Expansion of the digital cushion also causes the cushion to come into contact with the collateral cartilages, transferring the remainder of the force to the cartilages. The venous system of the collateral cartilage then

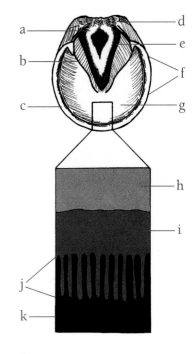

a: frog
b: bar
c: hoof wall
d: heel bulb
e: cleft of frog
f: quarter
g: sole
h: coffin bone
i: sensitive laminae
j: interdigitation of sensitive and insensitive laminae
k: hoof wall

1.4 The ground surface of the hoof. A cross section of the coffin bone, wall, and connecting laminae is shown.

---

1 Because of its location on the leg, the carpus appears similar to the human knee and is frequently referred to as the knee by horse owners and trainers. However, anatomically and functionally, the carpus is actually equivalent to the human wrist. The stifle is the true knee on a horse.

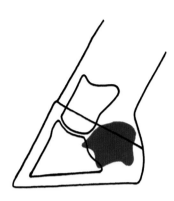

1.5 Position of the *lateral* collateral cartilage (in blue) of the hoof as viewed from the side of the horse. Each foot has two collateral cartilages—one on the medial aspect and one on the lateral aspect of the hoof.

absorbs the energy like the fluid of an automobile shock absorber. A similar action takes place at the coronary band venous network where the force that is transmitted up the hoof wall at contact is absorbed. Because of the changes to the venous network that occur during locomotion, the shock-absorbing functions of the foot act to maintain a healthy blood flow within the foot.

Hoof Care

The shock-dissipating system of the foot can function properly only if the foot is healthy. The hoof wall, sole, and frog must be well hydrated to maintain elasticity. The foot must be trimmed properly to allow the frog to contact the ground and the heels to expand. Balanced trimming of the foot is essential to even distribution of force over the shock-absorbing structures.

Daily Maintenance

The health of the hoof is a reflection of the health of the horse. Therefore, the best way to ensure a healthy foot is to maintain the horse's overall body condition. There are, however, horses that naturally have poor quality hoof walls that grow slowly and crack easily. Some of these horses can be helped by the addition of biotin, DL-methionine, and zinc to their diet. Biotin is a vitamin, DL-methionine is an amino acid, and zinc is a mineral. These are essential nutrients for hoof growth and are the main ingredient in many over-the-counter feed supplements formulated especially for maintenance of a healthy hoof.

The foot should be picked clean and examined daily. This not only helps prevent thrush (infection of the sole and frog), but also allows early identification of foreign bodies that may have become lodged in the foot. The foot should also be examined on a regular basis to identify developing imbalances.

Trimming the Foot

In general, Miniature horses have strong well-formed feet. The application of shoes is the exception rather than the rule. Whether the horse is barefoot or shod, maintaining hoof balance should be the main objective of the farrier. A foot is balanced when it is shaped so that the horse's weight is equally distributed over the foot when the horse is standing and the foot lands flat during motion.

When viewing a well-trimmed, balanced foot from the front, a line drawn through the coronary band is parallel to the ground and perpendicular to a line through the axis of the limb (fig. 1.6 A). When viewed from the side, the hoof wall at the toe is parallel to the slope of the heels and at the same angle as the pastern (fig. 1.6 B). When viewed from the rear, the heel bulbs are the same height, and when the foot is lifted off the ground, a line through the heel bulbs is perpendicular to the long axis of the limb (fig. 1.6 C). A balanced foot will impact the ground flatly when the horse is in motion.

Obviously, this description of balance is the ideal and is not attainable in every horse. When a horse's imbalance is a result of a conformation fault higher in the leg, trimming the foot to correct this imbalance may lead to lameness in the upper limb. In other cases, trimming to a perfect balance when the horse is standing results in a non-flat landing pattern. In these horses, consultation between the trainer, farrier, and veterinarian is often necessary to determine what trimming approach is most beneficial. **Radiographs** (X rays) of the feet are sometimes required to see the exact alignment of the bones of the leg in response to different trimming changes.

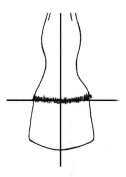

1.6 A A balanced foot as viewed from the front of the horse.

Trimming should be done every four to eight weeks. The length of time between trimmings depends on the rate of growth of the horse's foot and the amount of wear that occurs. Even if there is minimal growth of the foot, correction of imbalances that have developed since the previous trimming may be necessary. Therefore, trimming frequency should be tailored to each particular horse's needs.

The two most common hoof imbalances encountered in the Miniature horse are the overly high hoof angle and medial to lateral imbalance. When overly upright, the feet develop a boxy appearance. This type of foot loses some of its shock-absorbing capacity due to the lack of frog contact with the ground and its decreased ability to expand. In severe cases, a **club foot** may develop where the hoof wall at the toe is vertical to the ground or even tilts forward (see *Flexural Deformities,* p. 15). This type of foot results from excessive tension on the coffin bone from the deep digital flexor tendon, and may require surgical correction if trimming changes do not correct the imbalance.

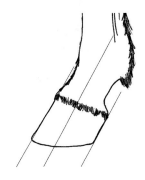

1.6 B The pastern angle, the hoof wall at the toe, and the hoof wall at the heels should all be parallel.

Medial to lateral imbalances cause the foot to turn in or out; the hoof rotates toward the longer wall (fig. 1.7). This can be due to improper trimming or rotation higher up in the limb. It is important to determine the origin of the imbalance, as trying to correct a rotated leg with aggressive trimming can result in a lame horse.

Hoof Diseases and Injuries

Puncture Wounds of the Foot
Puncture wounds of the foot are not unique to Miniature horses. However, because of the small size of their hooves, foreign objects can more easily penetrate deeper structures of the foot.

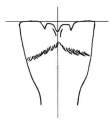

1.6 C A balanced foot seen when the foot is lifted.

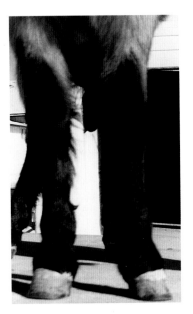

1.7 Outward rotation of both front feet. Notice that the carpi (known as "knees" in layman terms—see footnote, p. 5) are also rotated outward. It is unlikely that trimming changes will improve the rotation, as the source of the deformity is high in the leg.

CAUSE

The most common causes of puncture wounds of the foot are nails or other sharp objects that have been left in the horse's environment. The objects will initially catch on the sole or frog, then become more deeply imbedded as the horse walks.

DIAGNOSIS

Penetrating foreign objects of the sole or frog are generally discovered as part of daily hoof care or when the foot is examined because the horse becomes lame. The degree of lameness varies. If the object enters the sensitive tissues of the foot, the horse will be immediately lame. If the foot is entered at an oblique angle so that only the insensitive tissues are affected, lameness will not be evident unless infection develops at the site of penetration.

TREATMENT

The immediate reaction of most owners on seeing a nail entering the foot is to remove it when, in reality, this is the worst course of action. Determining the direction and depth of the puncture is critically important. Therefore, the nail should be left in place until a veterinarian examines the foot. In those cases where movement by the horse would drive the nail further into the foot, a wooden block can be applied to the foot with duct tape to prevent the horse from putting weight on the nail.

Radiographs may be taken to determine the exact course of the nail before it is removed (fig. 1.8). If the radiographs indicate that the navicular **bursa**, deep digital flexor **tendon sheath**, or coffin joint has been penetrated, the treatment and prognosis are very different from a simple puncture wound to the sole or frog.

The veterinarian's first line of treatment of a puncture wound is to open the foot to allow drainage of the infection. The nail is removed and the entrance hole enlarged with a hoof knife. This process is called "saucerizing the hole." Again, it is important that the nail be left in place until the veterinarian is available to treat the puncture wound. The sole and frog close over the defect quickly after removal of the nail, making the entrance hole nearly invisible within a few minutes. A tetanus booster should be given as soon as possible after the puncture has occurred.

Once a drainage route has been established, the foot should be soaked in Epsom salts for several days to draw the infection from the foot, and kept bandaged until the defect in the sole has completely healed. Lameness that occurs several days after the puncture has occurred is most likely due to an abscess developing at the puncture site. When this occurs, the abscess should be opened and drained followed by more soaking and bandaging of the foot until it heals.

If the veterinarian determines that the injury involves the joint, bursa, or tendon sheath, much more aggressive treatment is necessary. Infection of any of these structures can result in permanent, crippling lameness. These structures are fluid-filled, closed systems that make an ideal environment for bacterial growth. The blood supply to these areas is poor, limiting the effectiveness of oral, intravenous, and intramuscular antibiotics. Infection of the joint can lead to irreparable cartilage damage and severe arthritis. The result of infection in the bursa or tendon sheath is the formation of scar tissue (**adhesions**) to the deep digital flexor tendon that results in **chronic** pain. In addition, the navicular bone and the cartilage covering it will degenerate in the face of ongoing infection.

When a foreign object has entered the coffin joint, copious flushing of the joint with sterile fluid should be performed followed by placement of antibiotics directly into the joint. This is most effectively done under general anesthesia, and repeat treatments are necessary. If infection becomes established, an indwelling catheter that allows continuous input of antibiotics may be inserted into the joint. In the most severe cases, the joint may have to be surgically explored to allow removal of all infected tissue and drainage of the infection.

A surgical procedure called a street nail operation is performed when a foreign body penetrates the navicular bursa. A window is cut through the frog, digital cushion, and deep digital flexor tendon, into the navicular bursa. The bursa is flushed and infected tissue removed. The coffin joint and sheath of the deep digital flexor tendon are evaluated at the time of surgery, as spread of the infection into these areas is possible. These structures are also flushed if infection is suspected. The window is left open to allow drainage and further trimming of infected tissue, as necessary. The foot is bandaged until the defect completely heals.

PROGNOSIS

Simple puncture wounds to the sole or frog that do not involve the deeper structures of the hoof generally heal without incident. In those cases where an abscess forms at the puncture site, healing will usually occur without complication once the abscess is opened and drained.

Puncture wounds that enter the coffin joint, tendon sheath, or navicular bursa have a much poorer prognosis for future soundness. For example, in one report of twelve horses with infection in the coffin joint, only four horses became sound enough to be turned out to pasture and only one horse became

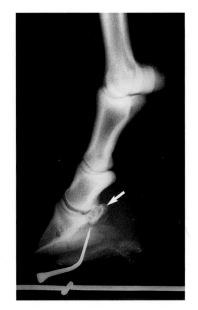

1.8 A radiograph of a nail puncture to the foot in the frog area. The radiograph reveals that the nail extends to the base of the navicular bone (the upper border of the navicular bone is marked with an arrow), entering the navicular bursa. The nail appeared to be heading away from the navicular area when examing the bottom of the foot, so without the radiographs, contamination of the navicular bursa would not have become apparent until the infection was well established.

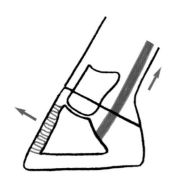

1.9 A The normal position of the coffin bone in the hoof wall as viewed from the side. The coffin bone is held in position against the pull of the deep digital flexor tendon (pictured in green) by the support of the interdigitating laminae that connect the coffin bone to the hoof wall (pictured in red). Note that the coffin bone is nearly parallel to the hoof wall and the ground surface.

sound enough for riding.[2] The most common cause of persistent lameness was arthritis that developed secondary to cartilage damage from the infection.

In a report on thirty-eight horses with puncture wounds to the navicular bursa, only twelve had a satisfactory outcome.[3] The best possible outcome was obtained when the street nail procedure was performed within one week of the puncture wound, before infection became well established. Complications seen secondary to the puncture wound included infection of the navicular and coffin bones, navicular bone fracture, and adhesions between the navicular bone and deep digital flexor tendon. Adhesions between the navicular bone and deep digital flexor tendon prevent normal range of motion of the tendon resulting in a mechanical lameness and painful stretching and tearing of the adhesion when the horse moves. While any of these complications may develop even if the surgery is performed immediately after the injury, the chance of complications greatly increases the longer surgery is delayed.

Quittor

The collateral cartilages can be infected secondary to a puncture wound or laceration. If a section of the cartilage becomes infected, a chronic draining tract called a **quittor** will develop.

DIAGNOSIS

A quittor is most commonly located at the coronary band near the heel. Because of this, it is sometimes confused with a **gravel** (a hoof wall abscess that opens and drains at the coronary band). The differences between the two are that a horse is usually very lame before a gravel breaks open whereas only mild lameness is seen with a quittor. Also, there is usually a history of a laceration or puncture wound with a quittor. Finally, a gravel will heal fairly quickly after it drains, whereas a quittor will continue to drain until the infected collateral cartilage is removed. A metal probe can be placed in the tract and followed to the collateral cartilage for a definitive diagnosis.

TREATMENT

Treatment consists of surgical removal of all infected cartilage. A hole is then created in the hoof wall to provide drainage to the area. The foot and the incision are kept bandaged until the surgery sites completely heal.

2 Honnas CM, Welch RD, Ford TS, Vacek JR, Watkins JP. Septic arthritis of the distal interphalangeal joint in 12 horses. *Vet Surg* 1992;21:261.

3 Richardson GL, O'Brien TR, Pascoe JR, Meagher DM. Puncture wounds of the navicular bursa in 38 horses. A retrospective study. *Vet Surg* 1986;15: 156

A good outcome can be expected if all the infected cartilage is removed and the foot receives appropriate care postoperatively.

Laminitis (Founder)

Laminitis, also known as **founder,** is a very painful condition caused by inflammation of the laminae that connect the hoof wall to the coffin bone. Many Miniature horse owners have the mistaken impression that Miniature horses cannot be affected by laminitis. While Miniatures seem more resistant to the disease than full-sized horses, laminitis does occur in Miniature horses and can result in a chronic, severe lameness.

In the early stages of laminitis, there is swelling and edema of the laminae secondary to either a decrease in the blood flow to the laminae or an influx of enzymes from the bowel that cause breakdown of the connections between the laminae. Because the swelling takes place in the confining wall of the hoof, a great deal of pain is associated with inflammation of the laminae. One can imagine the pain is similar to that experienced when a blood blister forms underneath a fingernail.

As the laminitis progresses, there is further degeneration of the laminae and separation of the coffin bone from the hoof wall. As the coffin bone separates from the wall, its position in the hoof will change. The toe may rotate downward due to the pull of the deep digital flexor tendon that attaches on the underside of the coffin bone near the toe (figs. 1.9 A & B). In very severe cases, the laminae are so damaged that the coffin bone will drop in the hoof as opposed to rotating. This drop of the coffin bone in the hoof wall is called "sinking."

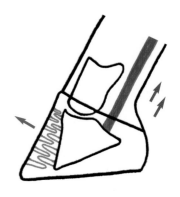

1.9 B The position of the coffin bone in a laminitic foot as viewed from the side. The laminae have started to degenerate and have lost their ability to support the coffin bone against the pull of the deep digital flexor tendon. As a result, the coffin bone is beginning to rotate within the hoof wall.

CAUSES

There are many possible causes for laminitis. These include obesity, overuse on a hard surface (road founder), overexposure to grass (grass founder), rapid change in diet, accidental over-ingestion of grain (grain founder), exposure to black walnut shavings or trees (contains a toxin that causes laminitis), administration of steroids, retained placenta, fever, diarrhea, overuse of a leg (for example, when the opposite leg has been injured and is too painful to bear weight), and **Cushings disease** (see *Cushings Disease,* p. 85). In addition, there are cases in which no predisposing cause for the laminitis can be seen.

DIAGNOSIS

Usually only the front feet are affected in laminitis, but in rare cases all four feet or only the rear feet may be involved. When the front feet are affected, the horse walks slowly and painfully, shifting its weight to the back feet,

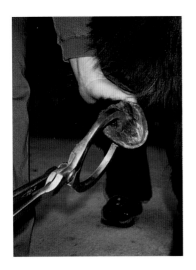

1.10 Hoof testers being applied to locate sensitive areas in the foot.

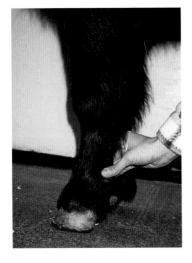

1.11 Digital pulses can be felt by putting gentle pressure on the digital arteries as they pass medially and laterally over the back of the fetlock.

especially when turning. Shifting weight back and forth between the rear feet may be an indication of rear limb laminitis. A severely affected horse may be unwilling to move, pick up its feet, or even stand.

A diagnosis of laminitis is made based on the movement of the horse, painful response to hoof testers over the soles (fig. 1.10), increased pulses to the foot, which is an indicator of inflammation (fig. 1.11), and radiographic changes (fig. 1.12). Rotation, or sinking of the coffin bone, is easily seen on radiographs, which help the veterinarian determine the course of treatment and establish a prognosis. In the early stages, there may be no evidence of rotation of the coffin bone. This can change during the course of the disease, so repeat radiographs are often necessary.

TREATMENT

The goal of treatment is to relieve the horse's pain and to prevent rotation or sinking of the coffin bone. There are many different approaches to this and none of the procedures are effective on all cases all of the time. Often, it is a matter of trying different treatments until an effective one is found.

The first step, when laminitis is suspected, is to confine the horse in a small area that is deeply bedded in straw or shavings. If separation of the laminae is occurring, every step that the horse takes will hasten that separation. The deep bedding will help keep the horse comfortable and take some of the stress off of the hoof wall. The use of frog support pads, which take the weight off of the horse's sole and wall, or Styrofoam pads taped onto the bottom of the horse's foot, are other ways of protecting the foot while making the horse more comfortable.

The mainstay of treatment is the use of **nonsteroidal anti-inflammatory drugs (NSAIDs)**. The most frequently used are *phenylbutazone* and *flunixin meglumine* (Banamine®). The action of these drugs is to decrease the inflammation of the laminae. This helps to slow or even stop the separation of the laminae and at the same time provides pain relief to the patient. The potent, pain-relieving effects of these drugs can mask the ongoing progression of the disease. Therefore, confinement and aggressive treatment for laminitis must be continued even if the horse shows great improvement when on the NSAIDs.

Careful dosing of NSAIDs is critical in Miniature horses. Overdosing can result in ulceration of the stomach (fig. 1.13), ulceration of the colon, or kidney failure. A single dose of *phenylbutazone* must never exceed 0.5 grams and the maximum dose of *flunixin meglumine* is 125 mg. These doses are for adult Miniature horses weighing 200–250 pounds (90–115 kg) and must be decreased further in foals and smaller Miniatures. The maximum dose must not be used for more than three days in adults and more than one day in foals. The safest approach to the use of NSAIDs is to use them only under the supervision of a veterinarian.

Another treatment that is applied with varying levels of success is drugs that improve the circulation in the foot including *isoxuprine, acepromazine,* and *nitroglycerine.* Isoxuprine is an oral drug that causes vasodilation (expansion of the blood vessels) and was developed to treat heart disease in people. It is frequently used in horses to increase blood flow to the foot in cases of laminitis and navicular disease. *Acepromazine* is a sedative that also causes vasodilation. Some horses show significant improvement when it is given orally or intramuscularly in cases of laminitis. Nitroglycerine cream is applied directly over the blood vessels on the back of the pastern. Its action is to dilate these vessels, thereby improving the blood flow to and out of the foot. Again, some horses seem to be helped by these treatments, while others show no significant improvement.

Corrective trimming and shoeing are used in almost all cases of laminitis. In the early stages of the disease before rotation has occurred, the use of wedges to raise the heel may help prevent rotation by relieving some of the pull of the deep digital flexor tendon. In chronic cases where rotation has already occurred, this may cause the horse more pain due to increased pressure on the sole. In all cases, any flaring of the toe of the foot should be removed and the hoof wall trimmed at the toe (without removing any weight-bearing wall or sole) to help decrease pull on the laminae, to make it easier for the foot to roll over the toe when the horse walks, and to encourage realignment of the hoof wall with the coffin bone when rotation is already present.

When rotation or sinking of the foot continues despite aggressive medical therapy, cutting of the deep digital flexor tendon is sometimes performed. The theory behind this procedure is to eliminate the pull on the coffin bone by the tendon. Once the pull has been eliminated, the shifting of the coffin bone should cease. This is a fairly drastic procedure and is generally used only in cases of laminitis that do not respond to medical treatment.

Important points for owners to be aware of when treating laminitis are:

- There are numerous approaches to fighting this disease.
- Each case should be assessed on an individual basis with all decisions on treatment made after evaluation by a veterinarian.
- Consultation between the veterinarian and farrier is vital to a successful outcome.
- It is not unusual for multiple treatments to be used before one is found that improves the horse's condition.

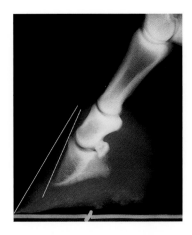

1.12 A radiograph of a Miniature horse with laminitis. Normally the coffin bone and hoof wall are parallel. This horse is affected with about 5 degrees of rotation.

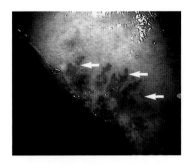

1.13 An **endoscopic** view of the inside of the stomach of a Miniature horse that was being treated for lameness with *phenylbutazone*. The red, irritated areas are gastric ulcers caused by the prolonged use of the drug.

- This is an extremely frustrating disease to treat. Some horses do not respond to any treatment and must be humanely destroyed because of continuous, unrelenting pain.
- If a horse does respond to treatment, it is prone to recurrence of the disease and must always be managed carefully to help prevent a relapse.

PROGNOSIS

The prognosis for future soundness after laminitis depends on the duration and severity of the disease. Many cases that are diagnosed and treated quickly, before rotation occurs, will respond well to treatment. Evidence of rotation on radiographs markedly decreases the chance for return to soundness, and the poorest prognosis is seen when sinking of the coffin bone is present. It is important for owners to realize that even if a horse makes a complete recovery, it will be more susceptible to future episodes of laminitis.

A study of 91 full-sized horses with laminitis was performed to determine the relationship between coffin bone rotation and future soundness.[4] Horses with less than 5.5 degrees of rotation had a favorable prognosis for future athletic use. The prognosis became guarded with rotation between 6.8 and 11.5 degrees, and horses with greater than 11.5 degrees of rotation had an unfavorable prognosis for athletic soundness. Some of the horses with greater than 11.5 degrees of rotation did become sound enough to be used for breeding. No such research has been performed in Miniature horses, but the study demonstrates the importance of preventing rotation through aggressive treatment at the first signs of the disease.

PREVENTION
- The best approach to laminitis is to do everything possible to prevent it.
- Do not allow any horse to become obese.
- Do not bed on shavings that contain any black walnut or allow access to black walnut trees.
- Make all changes in diet gradually, including the introduction to pasture in the spring.
- Keep grain behind locked doors and seek veterinary care immediately if a horse accidentally consumes more than the normal amount.
- Use steroids only under the guidance of a veterinarian.
- Maintain feet in good condition by regular trimming.

---

4 Stick JA, et al. Pedal rotation as a prognostic sign in laminitis of horses. *J Am Vet Med Assoc* 1982; 180: 251

- Closely monitor body temperature when a horse is sick and consult with the veterinarian whenever the temperature is above 101F (38C).
- Call a veterinarian if a mare does not pass her placenta within three hours of foaling.
- Finally, contact a veterinarian at the first signs of foot pain in a horse, as early treatment may prevent a minor case from turning into a catastrophic one.

Abnormalities of Growth

Flexural Deformities

Flexural deformities are conformational abnormalities that can be seen from the side of the horse, and are either *laxities* or ***contractures*** (figs. 1.14 A–G). A *laxity* is overextension of a joint caused by weakness of the tendons and ligaments that support the joint (figs. 1.14 B–D). Laxities of the lower limb are referred to as digital **hyper**extensions.

A *contracture* is excessive flexion of a joint caused by tightness of the supporting tendons and ligaments (fig. 1.14 E–G). One or more legs may be affected and a single joint or multiple joints may be involved in the deformity. The deformity may be **congenital** (present at birth) or **acquired** (develops over time).

The flexor tendons and suspensory ligament are the structures most frequently implicated in causing flexural deformities, although joint structures such as the joint capsule, also play a role in the laxity or contracture. The flexor tendons run down the back of the leg (blue and green lines in figs. 1.14 A–G). They function to bend the joints of the leg when the horse moves and support the back of the leg when the horse is standing. The suspensory ligament runs down the back of the cannon bone and acts to support the fetlock joint by preventing hyperextension of the joint during weight-bearing (red line in figs. 1.14 A–G).

Laxities

CAUSES

Common causes of *carpal laxity* and *digital hyperextension* in **neonates** (newborn foals less than 28 days of age) are premature birth or twinning. The cause of laxities in full-term, otherwise healthy foals is not known but may be related to disease in the mare, improper nutrition of the pregnant mare, or genetic predisposition.

1.14 A–G Flexural deformities
of the forelimb. The contributing
tendons and ligaments are
drawn for each deformity. A
dotted line is used to indicate
when the tendon or ligament
passes behind a bone on the
drawing. Blue: *flexor carpi ulnaris*
and *flexor carpi lateralis*. Green:
superficial digital flexor tendon.
Red: *suspensory ligament.*
Orange: *deep digital flexor
tendon.*

A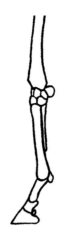

B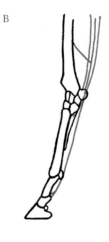

C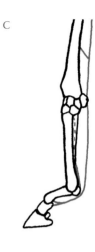

D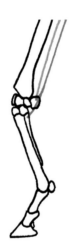

E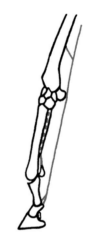

F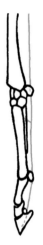

G

A Normal alignment of the
   bones of the forelimb.
B Laxity of the carpal joint.
C Laxity of the fetlock joint.
D Laxity of the coffin joint.
E Carpal joint contracture.
F Fetlock joint contracture.
G Coffin joint contracture.

DIAGNOSIS

Laxities are caused by a lack of support from the flexor tendons and/or suspensory ligament and are most commonly seen in newborn foals. The superficial flexor tendon and the suspensory ligament are the main support for the fetlock. When these are lax, the fetlock will drop and may even touch the ground (fig. 1.14 C), which in some cases can result in skin lesions on the back of the fetlock. Weakness in the flexor tendons may also contribute to carpal laxity (fig. 1.14 B). The main support to the hoof is the deep digital flexor tendon. When this tendon is lax, the toe of the foot will come off the ground (fig. 1.14 D).

TREATMENT

Carpal laxities and digital hyperextension in neonatal foals are due to lack of strength in the flexor tendons or suspensory ligament. Mild cases usually resolve in a few days to a few weeks as the foal grows and these structures become stronger. During this time, the mare and foal should be confined to a stall or small paddock. Confinement prevents over fatigue that may occur if the foal is forced to follow its mother in a large area. Any excess or pointy toe should be removed to encourage even breakover of the foot (figs. 1.15 A & B). Assisted swimming has been advocated as an effective form of physical therapy for these youngsters. The foal is supported in a swimming pool as it paddles about. The paddling action increases the strength of the supporting soft tissues without putting excessive strain on the limbs.

Caution: *It is critical that leg bandages or splints not be applied to a foal with digital hyperextension.* These devices take over the support of the limb, resulting in further weakening of the tendons and ligaments. If the skin needs to be protected, small, adhesive-type bandages can be placed over the wounds.

If the laxity worsens, does not resolve in a few weeks, or leads to sores from the foal's skin touching the ground, extensions can be added to the foot to support the limb. Heel extensions force the foal's toes onto the ground and help lift the fetlock. Extension can be accomplished by the use of glue-on shoes or acrylic augmentation to the hoof.[5] Small sections of wood or even tongue depressors can be taped to a Miniature horse foal's foot until a farrier or veterinarian can apply a more permanent support system (figs. 1.16 A–C). If glue-on shoes are used, they should be replaced

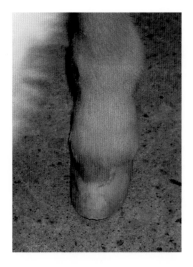

1.15 A A pointy toe on a five-day-old Miniature horse.

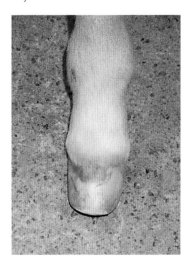

1.15 B The toe can be gently rounded with a rasp to encourage normal breakover at the center of the toe.

---

5 The #1 Ibex Babi-Cuff glue-on shoe will fit most Miniature horse foals and can be purchased through The Farrier and Hoofcare Resource Center. See Appendix D. An excellent description of the application of acrylic extensions by Steven E. O'Grady, DVM is available at www.equipodiatry.com. Click on "How to" then "create a Medial/Lateral Extension for Foal". The same technique is used to create toe and heel extensions. See Appendix D.

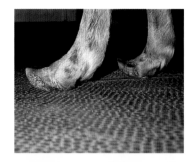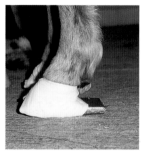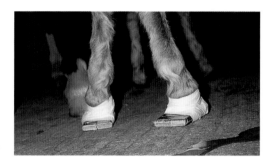

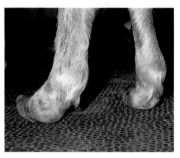

1.16 A (two views, above) A one-month-old Miniature filly with laxity of the deep digital flexor tendon.

1.16 B (two views, above right) The same filly with wooden supports taped to her feet.

often and removed as soon as possible to prevent contraction of the foot from confinement by the shoe. Glue-on shoes and acrylic wedges may become dislodged and have to be reapplied if the laxity has not resolved. As the foal gains strength, the size of the extensions can be gradually decreased and eventually removed.

In rare instances, the laxity will not correct as the foal ages. This syndrome is most commonly seen in **dwarf** Miniature horses (see Ch. 9, fig. 1). In addition to flexural laxity, the feet will often roll in or out, suggesting a weakness of the ligaments that support the inside and outside of the limb. There are several ways to manage these horses. The first is to continue to use heel extensions throughout the horse's life. If there is inward rolling of the feet, the outside wall must also be supported with an extension. An extension must also be applied to the inside of the hoof when there is an outward roll. Another option is a surgical procedure where the flexor tendons are shortened. This procedure does not correct the roll of the foot and must be combined with proper support for the hoof wall. Surgical fusion of the involved joints would eliminate both the flexural deformity as well as the roll of the foot. However, this complex surgical procedure is painful for the horse, requires extensive aftercare, and is expensive to perform.

PROGNOSIS

The majority of digital hyperextensions resolve in the first several weeks of life as the foal grows and becomes stronger. Cases of persistent laxity carry a poorer prognosis for resolution. Many of these horses must be indefinitely managed with heel extensions, or undergo surgical intervention to control the hyperextension.

Contractures

Contractural deformities are often referred to as contracted tendons when in fact the tendons are not contracted. Instead, the tendons are too short relative to the skeletal structure. Any number of legs may be affected, and any or all of the joints of the leg may be contracted. The most commonly affected joints are the carpal, fetlock, and coffin joints (see figs. 1.14 E–G). Contractures may be congenital (present at birth) or acquired (develop over time).

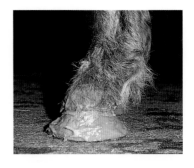

1.16 C
Acrylic has been applied to the filly's feet to provide additional heel support.

Congenital Contractures

CAUSES
Many contractural deformities are congenital. The cause of these deformities has not been determined but malpositioning in the mare, nutritional deficiencies of the mare during the pregnancy, and diseases acquired by the mare during pregnancy have been implicated.

DIAGNOSIS
Congenital contractures can be diagnosed easily by examining the newborn foal. Foals affected by contracture of the coffin joint walk on their toes (see fig. 1.14 G). If the contracture is located in the carpus, the joint will buckle forward (see fig. 1.14 E). Contractures of the fetlock range from a straight pastern-fetlock-cannon bone angle to buckling forward of the fetlock joint (see fig. 1.14 F). In severe contractures, the foal is unable to straighten the leg enough to stand.

TREATMENT
Treatment of congenital contractures depends on the affected joint and the severity of the abnormality. Some mild deformities can be corrected by simply bandaging the foal's legs. The bandages cause relaxation of the tendons. In more severe cases, application of splints or casts that force the leg into a normal position is the treatment of choice. Close monitoring of foals wearing splints or casts is vital, as the thin skin of the foal is very susceptible to pressure sores. Casts must be changed at least every ten days to prevent the cast from becoming too tight on the rapidly growing foal.

Applying glue-on shoes with toe extensions or acrylic toe extensions (see footnotes under *Laxity,* p. 17) may successfully treat foals with coffin joint contracture. The toe extensions help to stretch the deep digital flexor tendon each time the foal takes a step.

These treatments are often combined with intravenous administration of tetracycline. Tetracycline is an antibiotic that causes soft tissue relaxation. The exact mechanism of action is not known, but it has been shown to be effective in many cases.

In very severe cases, surgical intervention is necessary. Tendons and/or ligaments contributing to the contracture are cut (see *Treatment of Acquired Contractures,* p. 21). Sometimes, even this approach is not successful, and in

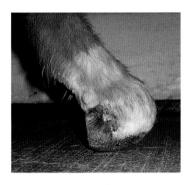

1.17 A severe *acquired* coffin joint contracture caused by lack of use of the limb due to a hip injury. The foot has rotated so that the sole is pointing backward, the horse is walking on the hoof wall, and the hoof is growing into the skin of the fetlock.

these cases, it is believed that the deformity is caused by tightness of the joint capsule itself. The prognosis for these foals is very poor and euthanasia may be the kindest action for them.

PROGNOSIS

The prognosis for correction of congenital contractures can be determined by manually attempting to straighten the leg. If correct, or nearly correct positioning of the joints can be obtained, the foal has a good chance of being treated successfully. If the joints cannot be straightened, successful treatment is unlikely.

Acquired Contractures

CAUSES

Acquired deformities are not present at birth, but develop over time. There are several possible causes of contractures developing in the growing foal. In rapidly growing foals, the ability of the tendons to elongate may not be equal to the rate of growth of the bone. Nutritional imbalances may contribute to the growth spurts or may be a primary cause of the contracture. Pain may also lead to contraction in a foal as well as an adult horse. When a limb is not used because of a painful condition, the muscles and tendons contract, leading to a flexural deformity (fig. 1.17). Overuse of a normal limb because of pain in the opposite limb can cause the previously normal limb to contract.

DIAGNOSIS

Acquired carpal and fetlock contractures can be diagnosed by visualization of the limbs. The carpus will buckle forward when contracted (see fig. 1.14 E). As in *congenital* contractures, *acquired* fetlock contractures can range from a straight pastern-fetlock-cannon bone angle to buckling forward of the fetlock joint (see fig. 1.14 F).

Because the appearance of the hoof wall can be misleading, acquired coffin joint contractures are best diagnosed using radiographs. The coffin bone on a normal horse will be in alignment with the pastern bones (fig. 1.18 A). The coffin bone is abnormally vertical in a horse with an acquired coffin joint contracture (fig. 1.18 B). In most cases, the hoof wall will also be overly upright. This conformation is referred to as a club foot. In severe cases, the coffin bone and hoof wall are tilted forward with the heel elevated off the ground (fig. 1.18 C).

Acquired coffin joint contractures have a different appearance than congenital contractures in that in congenital contractures, the foal walks on its toes, unable to place the heel on the ground. In all but the most severe acquired coffin joint contractures, the horse is able to place the heel on the ground, but the angle of the coffin joint and slope of the hoof wall has changed.

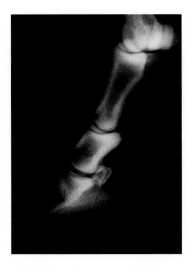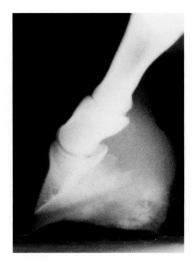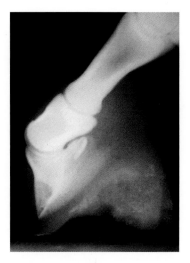

TREATMENT

The first course of treatment in cases of *acquired flexural deformities* is to attempt to determine and eliminate the primary cause. The first step is correction of nutritional deficiencies or imbalances. The entire feeding program should be analyzed, including nutritional analysis of the hay, in order to recognize and correct any deficits or excesses. Any lameness in young horses should be treated aggressively to prevent the formation of secondary flexural deformities.

Corrective trimming and shoeing are often successful treatments in acquired contractures if performed at the first signs of the deformity. Lowering the heels is used to treat coffin joint contracture and the use of toe extensions is helpful in both contractures of the coffin and fetlock joints. It is important that affected horses have regular, moderate exercise after the trimming, and that shoeing changes have been made to maximize the stretching of the flexor tendons.

As with congenital deformities, splints and casts may be applied in some cases of acquired deformities. Casts may be used for contracture of the carpus, fetlock, or coffin joint, but the use of splints is limited to carpal or fetlock contractures, as splints cannot be effectively applied to the coffin joint. It is important to closely monitor horses wearing these devices for early identification of pressure sores.

When these treatments are not effective, surgical intervention is necessary. Surgical treatment consists of cutting a ligament or tendon. What structure is cut depends on the location and severity of the contracture.

The preferred surgical approach to treating mild to moderate cases of *coffin joint contracture* (figs. 1.18 A & B) is to perform an *inferior check ligament*

From left to right

1.18 A A radiograph of a normal Miniature horse foot. Notice that the pastern bones and coffin bone are in near aligment.

1.18 B A Miniature horse with a mild acquired coffin joint contracture (club foot). Notice that the coffin bone forms an angle with the pastern and the hoof is more upright than normal. A successful outcome was obtained with an inferior check ligament desmotomy.

1.18 C A severe coffin joint contracture. This horse was treated successfully by cutting the deep digital flexor tendon.

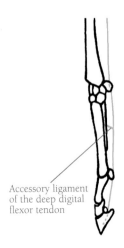

Accessory ligament
of the deep digital
flexor tendon

1.19 A The location of the accessory ligament of the deep digital flexor tendon. This diagram demonstrates a coffin joint contracture.

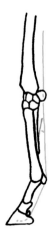

1.19 B The accessory ligament has been cut, allowing the deep digital flexor tendon to relax and the joint to return to a normal angle. Note: The red line shows where the surgical cut has been made.

desmotomy, a procedure where the accessory ligament of the deep digital flexor tendon is cut. The ligament originates on the bone under the carpus and attaches to the flexor tendon a short distance from its origin (fig. 1.19 A). It acts to provide support to the deep digital flexor tendon. When this ligament is cut, the flexor tendon is able to stretch, resulting in a decrease in the pull on the coffin bone (fig. 1.19 B). The ligament will eventually heal, but it will be longer than it was before surgery. Lowering of the heels and application of a toe extension are used in combination with the surgical procedure. This is a relatively simple surgery with good results in most cases. (It is also beneficial in some cases of *fetlock contracture.*)

When the coffin joint contracture results in a tilting forward of the hoof (see figs. 1.17 & 1.18 C), a more drastic approach must be taken. In this case, the deep digital flexor tendon itself must be cut (fig. 1.20). The post-operative recovery period is longer to allow the flexor tendon to heal. Weakness in the healed tendon can cause chronic lameness problems despite correction of the deformity.

Fetlock contractures can be treated by cutting the accessory ligament of the superficial digital flexor tendon, a procedure called a *superior check ligament desmotomy.* This ligament originates on the back of the **radius** (forearm) and attaches to the superficial digital flexor tendon above the carpus, giving additional support to the tendon (fig. 1.21 A). Cutting of this structure allows stretching of the superficial digital flexor tendon and relaxation of the fetlock contractures (fig. 1.21 B). Trimming and shoeing changes are made at the time of surgery and in more severe cases, a splint or cast is applied to put additional force on the contracture. A good outcome is usually obtained if the deformity is treated early; more chronic contractures do not respond as well to treatment. This procedure is performed in conjunction with cutting the accessory ligament of the deep digital flexor tendon in horses with a combination of contractures.

Mild cases of *acquired carpal contractures* may be successfully treated with splints or casts. If the application of splints or casts has failed to correct the deformity, two of the tendons that aid in flexion of the *carpus,* the *flexor carpi ulnaris* and *flexor carpi lateralis,* can be cut (figs. 1.22 A & B). Consistently good results have not been obtained with this surgery. While the surgery does not create any problems with the function of the carpus, it often does not completely correct the deformity.

PROGNOSIS

The prognosis for acquired fetlock contractures depends on the severity of the deformity. In mild cases, where the horse has a straight pastern-fetlock joint-cannon-bone angle, a successful outcome is likely. However, if the

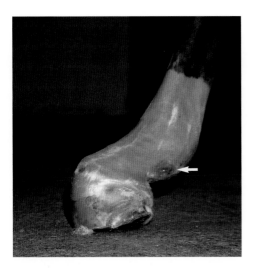

1.20 The immediate post-operative appearance of the horse shown in figure 1.17. Despite cutting the deep digital flexor tendon, the heel was unable to touch the ground after trimming the foot. The heel was purposely trimmed this short to encourage stretching of the coffin joint back to a more normal conformation. Note the wound on the back of the fetlock from where the hoof grew into the skin (see arrow).

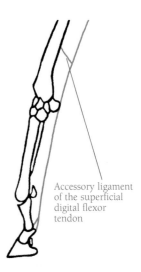

Accessory ligament of the superficial digital flexor tendon

1.21 A The location of the accessory ligament of the superficial digital flexor tendon. This diagram demonstrates a fetlock joint contracture.

fetlock buckles forward, complete correction, even with surgery, is unlikely.

Most cases of coffin joint contracture can be treated successfully. Many mild cases respond well to trimming and shoeing with toe extensions. In more severe cases where the hoof wall is nearly vertical, an inferior check ligament desmotomy is necessary, with a fair-to-good prognosis for resolution of the deformity and return to soundness postoperatively. When the hoof wall tips forward past vertical, the deep digital flexor tendon must be cut to resolve the contracture. While this procedure will likely correct the deformity, the deep digital flexor tendon will always be weaker than normal after healing. Therefore, the prognosis for future athletic soundness is guarded, but many Miniature horses become sound enough for light use.

In general, the prognosis for correction of acquired carpal contractures is guarded. Many cases cannot be straightened, even after surgical intervention. Fortunately, acquired carpal contractures are rare, and horses affected with carpal contracture remain sound even with athletic use if the contracture is not severe.

Angular Limb Deformities

Angular limb deformities (ALDs) are conformation abnormalities that can be viewed from the front of the horse (fig. 1.23). The carpi, hocks, or fetlocks can be involved and the deformity may be either congenital or acquired.

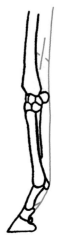

1.21 B The accessory ligament has been cut at the *red line*. This allows the superficial flexor tendon to relax and the joint to return to a normal angle.

1.22 A (left) A carpal contracture before surgical correction.

1.22 B (right) Cutting the *flexor carpi ulnaris* and *flexor carpi lateralis* tendons allowsthe carpus to return to a normal angle.

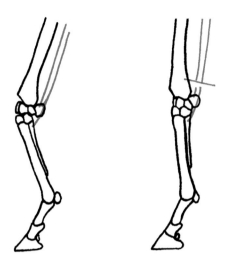

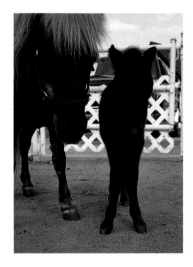

1.23 A five-day-old filly with an angular limb deformity (ALD) originating at the carpus. This ALD was due to periarticular laxity and resolved without treatment.

CAUSES

There are four possible causes of ALDs: laxity of the **periarticular** (surrounding the joint) structures that support the joint; collapse of incompletely formed bones in the carpus or hock (incomplete **ossification** of the **cuboidal bones**); growth plate abnormalities; and bridging of the **physis** by a complete **ulna** or **fibula**. These will be discussed in order.

Periarticular Laxity

Periarticular laxity is a common cause of ALDs in newborn foals and may be secondary to disease or improper nutrition of the pregnant mare, premature birth, or twinning. The soft tissues that support the joints (ligaments, joint capsule) are weak and do not provide adequate stabilization. As a result, the joint collapses when the leg is weight-bearing (fig. 1.23).

Incomplete Ossification of the Cuboidal Bones

An abnormality in the formation of the bones of the carpus or hock can also contribute to ALDs in these joints. The bones of these joints are called cuboidal bones because of their box-like shape (figs. 1.24 & 1.26). Like other bones in the body, these bones form in the developing fetus through a process called ossification.

The fetal precursor to bone is cartilage. As the fetus matures, the cartilage is gradually converted to bone. If a foal is a twin, is born prematurely, or some abnormal influence during fetal development slows the ossification process (disease or improper nutrition of the pregnant mare), the bones will not be completely formed at birth. This is called *incomplete ossification of the cuboidal bones* (fig. 1.24). Because cartilage is not as strong as bone, these

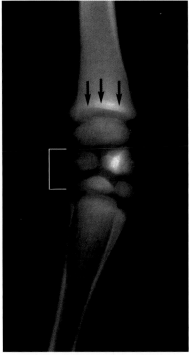

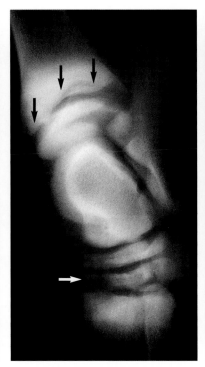

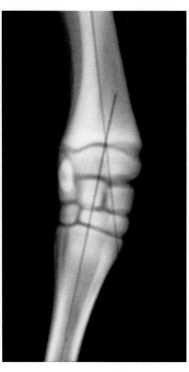

1.24 Incomplete ossification of the cuboidal bones of the *carpus*. The spaces between the immature bones are filled with cartilage that will gradually mature into bone (Compare this radiograph to figure 1.26 where the cuboidal bones of the carpus are completely ossified.) Note the angular limb deformity (ALD) putting pressure on the immature bones on the lateral aspect of the joint (white bracket), predisposing them to crushing. A splint or cast should be applied to this leg to support the carpus until ossification is complete. Black arrows mark the location of the radial physis (growth plate).

1.25 Incomplete ossification of the cuboidal bones of the *hock*. There is a evidence of crushing of the incompletely formed bones at the front of the hock (white arrow). The bones that replace the crushed cartilage will also be malformed, resulting in a sickle-hock conformation. As in Figure 1.24, a cast or splint should be applied until ossification is complete. The black arrows mark the location of the tibial physis (growth plate).

1.26 An angular limb deformity (ALD) of the carpus caused by asymmetric growth at the physis (growth plate). The medial aspect of the physis is growing more rapidly, resulting in a medial bowing of the leg (medial is to the right and lateral is to the left). Lines drawn through the long bones (radius above and cannon bone below) intersect at the physis, indicating that it is the source of the deformity. Two surgical options are available to correct this deformity. Growth acceleration (periosteal stripping can be performed on the slow-growing, concave (lateral side), or growth retardation (transphyseal bridging) can be performed on the fast-growing, convex (medial) side of the physis.

incompletely formed bones are at risk for crushing if stressed. If the cartilage crushes or collapses, the bones that replace the cartilage during the ossification process will also be crushed or collapsed, resulting in a permanent deformity that cannot be corrected.

In addition to causing ALDs, incomplete ossification of the cuboidal bones of the hock can also lead to crushing of the cartilage in the front of the hock joint (fig. 1.25). This results in a collapse of this section of the joint and a permanent sickle hock conformation (a conformational abnormality where the hock is excessively angulated as viewed from the side).

Growth Plate Abnormalities

The long bones increase in length by laying down new bone (ossification) at a growth plate (physis), an area of cartilage located near the end of the bone. The cartilage at the physis is replace by bone until growth is complete. Physes (plural for physis) are present in the long bones above the carpus, hock, and fetlock joints: at the end of the radii above the carpi (figs. 1.24, 1.26 & 1.27), at the end of the tibiae above the hocks (fig. 1.25), and at the end of the cannon bones above the fetlocks. Because cartilage is invisible on radiographs, the physis is easily identified on radiographs as an irregular black line near the end of the bone (figs. 1.24, 1.25 & 1.26).

Asymmetric growth at the physis will result in an ALD of the joint below it. If one side of the physis grows faster than the other, the leg will start to bow toward the fast growing side (fig. 1.26). This type of deformity may be present in newborn foals due to abnormal fetal growth, but frequently develops in the growing foal secondary to nutritional imbalances, excessive exercise, or trauma.

Complete Ulna or Fibula

In humans, two bones are present in the forearm: the radius and ulna. Similarly, two bones are present in the calf: the tibia and fibula. In horses, these bones are separated at the top of the leg, but fuse about halfway down the radius in the front leg and halfway down the tibia in the rear leg (see fig. 1.1). Therefore, in horses, the lower half of the forearm consists of one bone (the radius) and the lower half of the upper leg[6] consists of one bone (the tibia).

This final cause of ALDs is rare in full-sized horses, but not unusual in Miniature horses. In some Miniature horses, a *complete ulna or fibula* is present. When this occurs, the ulna or fibula runs the entire length of the radius or tibia, bridging the lateral aspect of the physis, preventing growth on that

---

6 The anatomic area on the horse that corresponds to the human calf lies between the stifle (equivalent to the human knee) and the hock (equivalent to the human ankle).

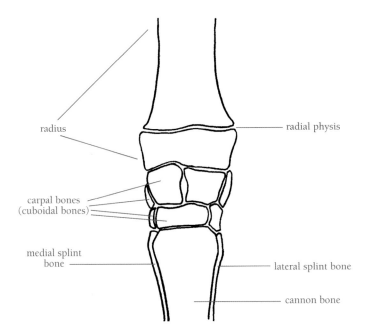

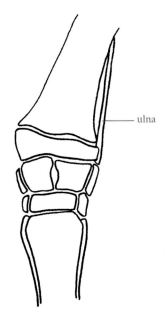

radius

radial physis

carpal bones
(cuboidal bones)

medial splint
bone

lateral splint bone

cannon bone

ulna

side (figs. 1.27 A & B). As a result, the leg begins to bow medially at the carpus or hock as the foal grows. This abnormality seems to be associated with dwarfism in Miniature horses.

DIAGNOSIS

Angular limb deformities are easily diagnosed with observation of the affected joint or joints. The important step in the diagnostic process is determining the cause of the deformity, as this will establish the treatment approach. To this end, manipulation and radiographs of the joint should be performed on all cases of ALDs.

Angular limb deformities caused by *periarticular laxity* are seen in newborn foals. Multiple joints are frequently affected and the ALD is often seen in conjunction with flexural laxity (see *Flexural Deformities,* p. 15). The affected joint can be manually straightened to a normal angle. In ALDs caused purely by periarticular laxity, the radiographs will be normal, but radiographs should be taken of any foal with periarticular laxity as many will also have incomplete formation of the cuboidal bones.

Like periarticular laxity, incomplete *ossification of the cuboidal bones* is seen in neonates and the affected joint can be manually straightened. The incompletely formed cuboidal bones are easily identified on radiographs (see fig. 1.24). Radiographs should be taken of any foal, whether full term or premature, that has an ALD of the carpi or hocks. Radiographs should

1.27 A (left) Normal anatomy of the equine carpus.

1.27 B (above) The abnormal presence of an ulna (long bone of the forelimb that normally fuses with the radius halfway down the forearm)in the carpus, which is bridging the physis (growth plate) and preventing growth on that side of the limb. The result is an angular limb deformity (ALD) with medial bowing of the leg. Surgical removal of the ulna is necessary to correct this deformity.

also be taken of any foal that is born prematurely or appears immature at birth, even if the foal's legs are straight.

Asymmetric growth at the physis of any joint can occur at any time during the first six months of life in Miniature horses. The ALD is frequently seen in combination with rotation of the limb and the leg cannot be manually straightened. Confirmation that the physis is the source of the deformity is made using radiographs. Lines are drawn along the center of the long bones of the affected leg, crossing the deformed joint. The point of intersection of the lines marks the origin of the deformity (see fig. 1.26). The radiographs will also demonstrate the presence of an ulna in the carpus or a fibula in the hock that may be contributing to the uneven growth.

TREATMENT

The first line of treatment of foals with ALD caused by periarticular laxity is stall rest with short periods of exercise. Before beginning exercise, the foal's feet should be filed to remove any excess or pointed toe (see fig. 1.15). Exercise should consist of five to ten minutes of walking beside the mare on a soft surface. It is important that the exercise be controlled as the conformation of the limbs puts abnormal stresses on the joints.

Caution: Radiographs must be taken before exercise is initiated in any foal with ALD or any premature or immature foal to rule out incomplete bone formation.

If the cuboidal bones are not completely formed, the foal should not be exercised. Assisted swimming is an excellent therapy for soft-tissue laxities with or without incomplete formation of the cuboidal bones. The advantage of swimming is that it strengthens the soft tissues without causing undue trauma to the joint.

Bandages should not be applied to foals with ALDs caused by periarticular laxity. Bandaging takes the stress off the supporting soft tissues, preventing them from strengthening.

Most simple periarticular laxities will resolve in the first week of life. If the ALD persists, the foal should be reevaluated after the first week to see if there are other factors contributing to the deformity. The use of glue-on shoes or acrylic extensions on the feet may help correct cases of persistent soft-tissue laxity. If the leg is bowing medially (inward), the extensions should be applied to the medial aspect of the hoof. If the leg is bowing out laterally (outward), the extensions should be applied to the lateral aspect of the hoof (see footnotes under *Laxity,* p. 17).

Angular limb deformities caused by persistent periarticular laxity is commonly seen in dwarf Miniature horses. Flexural laxity is usually present with the ALD in these horses (see *Flexural Deformities,* p. 15). Surgical fusion of the affected joints will eliminate the deformity and is a viable option in the lower joints of the limb. Fusion of the carpi or hocks is not practical, as the foal needs to flex these joints in order to ambulate.

When incomplete ossification of the cuboidal bones is identified on radiographs treatment depends on whether or not an ALD is present. If the legs are straight, the foal should be stall rested until the ossification process is complete. This may take as long as two months and radiographs are necessary to determine when the bones are completely formed. If a foal with incomplete ossification is allowed to exercise, crushing of the cuboidal bones is likely.

If the foal has an ALD along with incomplete ossification of the cuboidal bones, the leg is manually straightened and splints or casts applied to hold the limb in normal alignment, protecting the immature bones from the abnormal stresses of the deformity. The splints or casts are left in place until the bones have completely ossified, and should be changed frequently to check for pressure sores and to allow for the foal's growth.

The first step in treatment of foals with ALD due to asymmetric growth at the physis is to remove any excess hoof at the toe, and round the toe for an even breakover (see fig. 1.15). These foals should be confined to a stall to prevent overuse of the affected limb. In mild cases, this may be all that is needed to correct the ALD and the rotational deformity that frequently accompanies it. In more severe cases, the use of glue-on shoes or acrylic extensions is indicated. As with periarticular laxities, the extension is placed on the medial aspect of the hoof when the leg bows medially (inward), and on the lateral aspect when it bows laterally (outward).

If these treatments do not resolve the irregular growth, surgical corrections can be performed. In order to be successful, the deformity must be corrected while the foal is still rapidly growing. Miniature horse foals have less growth potential than full-sized horse foals. Therefore, surgical correction must be performed at a younger age. The growth plates of the fetlock are the most active during the first month of life. Surgical correction of ALDs in this joint must be completed before the foal is one-month old. Growth at the carpus and hock significantly decrease after four months; surgical correction of carpal and hock ALDs should be completed before the foal reaches this age.

There are two options for surgical correction of ALDs originating at a physis: *growth acceleration* or *growth retardation.* Growth acceleration is performed on the side of the physis that is demonstrating sluggish growth (the concave side). The covering of the bone (**periosteum**) is elevated from around the physis, stimulating growth on that side. Growth retardation is performed by placing a wire or plate across the physis on the side showing the more rapid growth (the convex side). This is called transphyseal

1.28 Anatomy of the stifle.

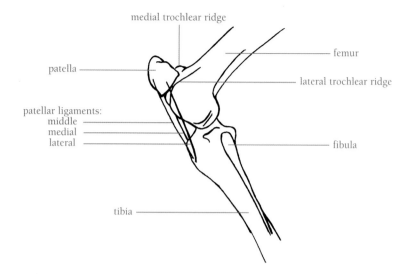

medial trochlear ridge

patella

patellar ligaments:
middle
medial
lateral

tibia

femur

lateral trochlear ridge

fibula

bridging: The wire or plate must be removed when correction of the deformity has been obtained.

Which procedure is used depends on the severity of the deformity and the age of the foal. If the foal is young and the deformity is mild, growth acceleration is often successful. If the deformity is severe or the foal is older, growth retardation is the treatment of choice. Growth retardation is combined with growth acceleration in moderate to severe deformities where there is little time left to correct the ALD. In these cases, transphyseal bridging is performed on the on the fast-growing side (convex) of the physis, and periosteal stripping performed on the slow-growing (concave) side of the physis.

When the ALD is caused by the presence of an ulna or fibula, surgical removal of the abnormal bone is necessary. Growth acceleration or growth retardation should be performed simultaneously to correct the deformity. Again, which procedure is used depends on the age of the foal and the severity of the deformity.

PROGNOSIS

Most cases of ALD can be corrected if treatment is initiated early. The exception is periarticular laxities that do not respond to treatment in the first several weeks of life. Many of these foals must wear supportive shoes, or hoof extensions, for the rest of their life or undergo surgical fusion of the affected joints.

Cases of incomplete ossification of the cuboidal bones will have a good outcome if the abnormality is identified before crushing of the cartilage precursor occurs. Once collapse of the cartilage has occurred, little can be done to correct the resulting ALD as the bone that forms will also be collapsed. Therefore, the importance of radiographs in any foal with an ALD of the carpus or hock, or any foal that is suspected of being at risk for incomplete ossification of the cuboidal bones, cannot be overemphasized.

The most frequent cause of failure in cases of ALD due to **physeal** abnormalities is delay of treatment until after the foal has passed its rapid growth phase. As I said earlier, if treatment is delayed past one month in fetlock deformities or past four months in carpal or hock deformities, surgical correction is unlikely to be successful.

There is ongoing debate on the ethics of surgical correction of ALDs. It is true that there may be a hereditary component to the deformity, especially in dwarf Miniature horses. For this reason, affected horses should be removed from the breeding pool. Many Miniature horses with mild deformities live comfortable lives and are able to stay sound as long as athletic performance is not required. However, severe deformities lead to chronic pain from arthritis and soft tissue strain (see fig. 9.1). If such a deformed animal is allowed to live, every attempt should be made to correct or improve the deformity so that the animal has a chance at a pain-free life.

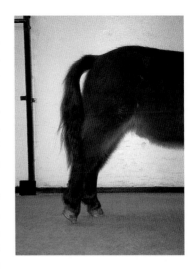

1.29 A typical appearance of an upward fixation of the patella (locking of the stifle). Notice that the leg is fixed in extension and the front of the hoof drags on the ground.

Patella Issues

Upward Fixation of the Patella

ANATOMY
Figure 1.28 shows the anatomy of the stifle, the equine equivalent of the human knee. When a horse moves, the patella (kneecap) slides up and down a groove in the end of the femur called the trochlear groove. The boundaries of the groove are two bony ridges called the medial and lateral trochlear ridges. The patella is stabilized in this groove by patellar ligaments that are attached to the quadriceps muscles.

DIAGNOSIS
Upward fixation of the patella, also called *locking of the stifle,* occurs when the patella catches on the top of the medial trochlear ridge. Upward fixation of the patella is easily recognized by the characteristic gait and stance of the affected horse. The leg becomes fixed in extension (extending behind the horse); the fetlock can flex, but the hock and stifle cannot (fig. 1.29). The front of the hoof will drag on the ground if the horse is forced to move forward. The fixation may correct itself only to lock again a few steps later.

Some horses may even stay locked for several hours or even days. Upward fixation of the patella can also occur sporadically, with the patella popping off the ridge without assistance, creating a catch in the horse's gait. This is called intermittent upward fixation of the patella.

CAUSES

Several causes of this condition have been described. There may be a hereditary predisposition to upward fixation of the patella as horses with a straight hind limb conformation are more commonly affected. The locking may also be caused by trauma when the leg is fully extended. Horses with poor muscle tone from lack of conditioning are predisposed. This is due to inability of the quadriceps muscles to tense the patella ligaments, an action that is necessary to control the motion of the patella.

TREATMENT

Treatment depends on the severity of the condition. Cases of intermittent upward fixation of the patella due to lack of muscle tone in the quadriceps are treated with physical therapy. Horses are placed on a steady routine of exercise to strengthen the quadriceps muscles. Walking up and down hills is an excellent strengthening exercise. Some veterinarians elect to augment this exercise program with injection of the patellar ligaments with an internal iodine blister. This causes scar tissue to form around the ligaments, increasing their stiffness. The theory behind this procedure is that laxity of the patellar ligaments allows a greater range of motion of the patella, predisposing the horse to upward fixation. Decreasing this range of motion would therefore decrease the likelihood of the fixation occurring.

In horses where the patella is completely trapped on the trochlear ridge, the first step in treatment is to unlock the stifle. This is accomplished by pushing downward and inward on the patella while pulling the leg forward or pushing the horse back. If the problem is due to trauma, this manipulation is often all that is needed to correct the problem. However, if the locking is due to a conformational abnormality, the upward fixation will likely recur, sometimes as soon as the horse takes another step. In these severe cases, surgical correction may be necessary.

Surgical correction of upward fixation of the patella consists of cutting the medial patellar ligament, thereby decreasing the inward pull on the patella. While this is very effective in correcting a locked stifle, it also results in instability of the patella. Degeneration of the cartilage of the patella and secondary arthritis is a potential complication of this instability. Therefore, it is recommended that surgical correction only be performed on those cases that do not respond to any other treatment.

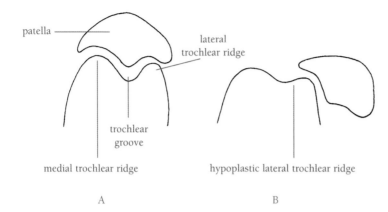

patella

lateral
trochlear ridge

trochlear
groove

medial trochlear ridge

hypoplastic lateral trochlear ridge

A

B

1.30 A diagram of a lateral luxation of the patella, looking down the femur at the stifle joint. A) Normal position of the patella in the trochlear groove of the femur. B) Lateral luxation of the patella due to hypoplasia of the lateral trochlear ridge. Notice how the lateral trochlear ridge is very flat and the trochlear groove is shallow.

PROGNOSIS

Horses affected with intermittent upward fixation of the patella due to poor tone of the quadriceps muscles respond well to exercise. However, recurrence of the problem is likely if the horse receives extended time off from its work schedule.

Unlike in full-sized horses where intermittent upward fixation that responds to exercise is the most common presentation of this abnormality, upward fixation of the patella in Miniature horses is frequently seen as complete locking that can only be corrected with surgery. There is a good prognosis for correction of this type of upward fixation of the patella with surgery, but the long term effects of the surgery in Miniature horses are not known. While the surgery commonly results in degeneration of the patella in full-sized horses, enough data is not available to identify how frequently this occurs postoperatively in Miniature horses.

Luxation of the Patella

Luxation of the patella is a disease where the patella becomes dislocated from its normal position in the stifle. Most frequently, it slips laterally out of its position in between the trochlear ridges to the outside of the stifle (fig. 1.30) although medial dislocation is possible. This condition can be seen in adult animals secondary to trauma, but more commonly, it is a congenital abnormality that is evident within the first few months of life. In congenital luxations, one stifle may be affected, but usually both stifles are involved. Congenital patellar luxation is more common in Miniature horses than in

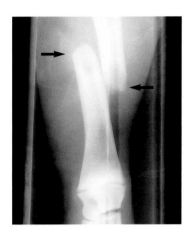

1.31 A A radial (forearm) fracture in a yearling Miniature horse. The overriding bone ends are marked with black arrows.

other breeds. In fact, the majority of cases reported in the veterinary literature have been in Miniature horses.

There are two possible causes of patellar luxation—*trauma,* and *lateral trochlear ridge* **hypoplasia.** Traumatic patellar luxation occurs due to tearing of the supporting soft tissues of the medial aspect of the joint (the joint capsule and medial patellar ligament). This weakens the medial support of the patella, allowing it to shift out of the trochlear groove to the outside of the joint.

Lateral trochlear ridge hypoplasia is a congenital deformity where the lateral trochlear ridge is flatter and smaller than normal resulting in a shallow trochlear groove for the patella (fig. 1.30). The patella can then easily slip out of the groove to the outside of the joint. In some foals, tearing of the medial supporting soft tissues is seen in conjunction with lateral trochlear ridge hypoplasia, probably secondary to the lateral displacement of the patella.

DIAGNOSIS

Diagnosis of traumatic luxation of the patella is made based on the history of a recent injury followed by severe rear-limb lameness. The patella can be palpated (felt) sitting lateral to the stifle joint, and radiographs can be taken to confirm the diagnosis.

The clinical signs of lateral trochlear ridge hypoplasia depend on the severity of the condition. The foal may walk with a stiff gait, unwilling to bend the stifle. In severe cases, the foal may not be able to stand or can only stand for short periods of time with the stifle in a flexed position. Like traumatic luxation, the patella can be palpated sitting lateral to the stifle and radiographs are used to confirm the luxation. Radiographs are also useful to evaluate the degree of lateral trochlear ridge hypoplasia and to determine if secondary damage to the joint is present.

TREATMENT

Surgical correction of luxation of the patella is recommended. If the condition is not treated, severe, crippling arthritis will develop.

One approach to surgical treatment of lateral luxation of the patella is to perform a *lateral release of the patella* by partially cutting the tissues that support the outside of the joint. This relieves the lateral pull on the patella and allows it to slide back into its normal position. The lateral release is always combined with placement of tightening sutures on the medial aspect of the joint—a *medial imbrication.* The combination of the *lateral release* and *medial imbrication* will usually bring the patella back into the trochlear groove. This procedure is most successful if the trochlear ridges are normal.

The other surgical treatment is used when the luxation is due to severe flattening of the lateral trochlear ridge. In these cases, the trochlear groove in the femur is surgically deepened, a procedure called *trochleoplasty*. The cartilage is lifted from the bone, a section of bone removed, and the cartilage sutured back into place. This procedure is frequently combined with lateral release and medial tightening of the joint. Trochleoplasty is more difficult and has more complications than the lateral release procedure. Therefore, it is usually reserved for severe cases of lateral trochlear ridge hypoplasia or if a lateral release was not successful.

PROGNOSIS

The most common cause of failure of these surgeries is disruption of the repair and reluxation of the patella during recovery from anesthesia. This is less of a problem in Miniature horses because their small size results in less strain on the repair. In addition, while assisting large horses to stand after anesthesia is difficult and sometimes dangerous for the handlers, Miniature horses can easily be helped to their feet without the risk of injury to the people providing assistance. As a result, these surgeries carry a much better prognosis for success in Miniature horses. However, it is important that surgery be performed as soon as possible after the luxation has been diagnosed to decrease the risk of secondary arthritis.

Fractures

CAUSES

Like full-sized horses, Miniature horses can fracture any bone of the body. In large horses, *fractures* are usually a result of the forces that a horse applies to its own limbs. Examples of this are leg fractures in racehorses and fractures of the pastern that occur as a result of twisting forces produced in Western performance horses such as cutters and reiners. These types of fractures are rare in Miniature horses due to their small size and the type of work they perform. Miniature horse fractures are more frequently due to external trauma such as a kick.

TREATMENT

Some simple fractures can be treated with casting, but in most cases, maximum stability of the healing fracture is obtained with **internal fixation.** In internal fixation, various combinations of plates, screws, and wires are used to stabilize the fracture (figs. 1.31 A & B). The resulting stability not only speeds the healing of the fracture, but also allows the horse to be more comfortable during the healing process.

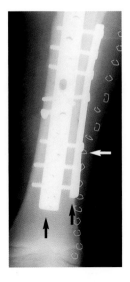

1.31 B The repair of the above fracture. Two plates with screws have been used to stabilize the fracture (black arrows). This type of fracture carries a poor prognosis in a full-sized horse, but this Miniature horse recovered completely. The oval metallic structures to the right of the bone (white arrow) are skin staples.

The success of the fracture repair depends on the condition of the bone ends and overlying soft tissues at the time of surgery. Therefore, a fracture patient must never be transported without proper support to the injured area. Ideally, a splint or cast should be applied to immobilize the limb. If this is not possible, a heavy bandage should be applied. Treatment for shock with intravenous fluids may also be necessary before transporting the animal to a surgical facility.

PROGNOSIS

Miniature horses have a huge advantage over full-sized horses when recovering from fractures. Their small size puts less stress on the healing bone. They are also less likely to breakdown in the opposite, weight-bearing limb, a common cause of euthanasia in large horses with fractures. Bending or breaking of internal fixation devices is a common cause of fixation failure in large horses, a complication rarely seen in Miniature horses. While the chance of a successful repair depends on the severity and location of the fracture, many fractures in Miniature horses can be repaired with a good prognosis for a sound animal.

Summary

There are numerous differences between Miniature and full-sized horses with respect to the musculoskeletal system. Lameness problems are relatively rare in Miniature horses; this is probably due to their small size and the type of work they perform. Many musculoskeletal abnormalities, such as patellar luxations and fractures, carry a much better prognosis for successful treatment than in full-sized horses. However, abnormalities that are related to growth, such as angular limb deformities (ALDs), must be addressed at an earlier age in Miniature horses, as they reach their growth potential sooner than full-sized horses.

CHAPTER 2

The Respiratory System

THE PRIMARY FUNCTION of the respiratory system is to provide oxygen to the blood. To accomplish this, air must pass through the nasal passageway, nasopharynx, and trachea to the lungs where oxygen diffuses through the thin walls into the bloodstream. Because the horse is primarily an athletic animal, there must be as little **impedance** to the flow of air as possible, especially during maximal exercise. The structures of the equine airway also play an important role in warming and cleaning the air that is delivered to the lungs, protecting the airway from aspiration of food, and cooling the air that is delivered to the brain.

Miniature horses can be affected by most of the respiratory abnormalities and all of the infectious respiratory diseases that affect full-sized animals. There are several respiratory abnormalities that require special attention with respect to treatment in Miniature horses.

The Structure and Function of the Respiratory Tract

Nasal Passages and Sinuses

The nasal passages start at the nostrils and end at the nasopharynx (fig. 2.1). Paired passages are separated by the nasal septum. The lining is filled with blood vessels that lie close to its surface. These blood vessels help to warm the air as it passes over them. The size of the nasal passage is much smaller than what is suggested by the size of the horse's head. This is because the teeth and sinuses take up much of the space of the head, limiting the size of the airway.

The sinuses are air-filled structures in the skull (fig. 2.2). The function of the sinuses is not known, but the weight of the head is markedly less than what it would be if the skull were solid bone. The sinuses communicate with the nasal passage through small drainage ports, allowing

2.1 The anatomy of the equine
upper respiratory tract.

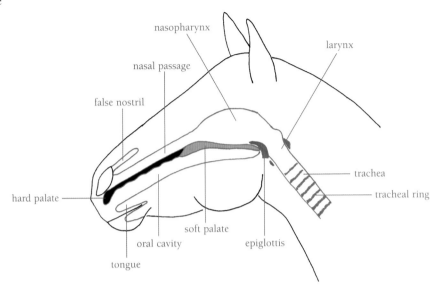

2.2 The location of the
maxilary sinus (red), frontal
sinus (blue), and guttural pouch
(green). These are paired structures, meaning that they are
located on both sides of the
skull, so that there are two
maxillary sinuses, two frontal
sinuses, and two guttural
pouches.

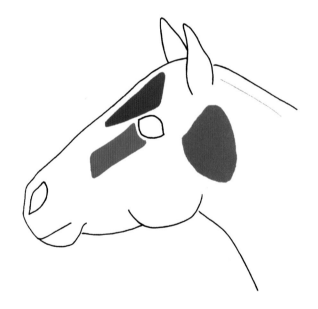

normal sinus secretions to pass out the nose. This drainage process is critical in preventing a buildup of fluid and bacteria in the sinus. The maxillary sinus is important in that the roots of the last four cheek teeth are located in this sinus. A very thin plate of bone separates the tooth roots from the sinus space.

Nasopharynx and Guttural Pouches

The nasal passages come together to form the nasopharynx, an enlargement of the upper airway directly in front of the entrance to the trachea. It is separated from the oral cavity by the soft palate (fig. 2.1). This separation is completed by the epiglottis, a triangular-shaped flap of cartilage that flips up in front of the opening of the trachea when the horse swallows, thereby protecting the airway from aspiration of food (figs. 2.1 & 2.3). The free margin of the soft palate lies underneath the epiglottis during respiration. For this reason, horses are obligate nose breathers; they are unable to breathe through their mouth, even under extreme respiratory stress.

The guttural pouches are large air-filled sacs that lie on either side of the head in the throatlatch area (fig. 2.2). The openings of the guttural pouches are located in the nasopharynx (fig. 2.4). The guttural pouches are enlargements of the eustachian tubes, tubes that run between the ear canal and nasopharynx (In humans, it is the presence of the eustachian tubes that allow a person to equalize pressure changes in their ears by swallowing during air travel.). The arteries that supply the brain pass through these large air-filled pouches. It is believed that the air present in the guttural pouches cools the blood on its way to the brain, preventing overheating of the brain during periods of heat stress, such as intense exercise in hot weather.

Larynx and Trachea

The larynx is located at the opening of the trachea and is made up of movable sections of cartilage, including the epiglottis (figs. 2.1 & 2.2). It closes when the horse swallows to protect the airway from food inhalation and opens wider in response to increased demand for air during exercise.

The trachea is a flexible, semi-rigid tube that extends from the larynx to the lungs. The rigidity of the trachea is provided by cartilage rings, which encircle the trachea. A strip of muscle (trachealis muscle) connects

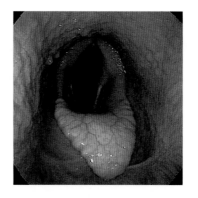

2.3 An endoscopic view of the larynx, the entrance to the trachea. The triangular shaped cartilage at the bottom of the photo is the epiglottis, which flips up to protect the airway when the horse swallows. The soft palate lies underneath the epiglottis.

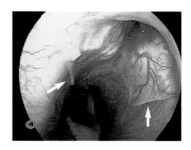

2.4 An endoscopic view of the nasopharnyx showing the location of the guttural pouch openings (slits marked by the arrows). Notice the larynx in the background and the large number of blood vessels running on the surface of the airway.

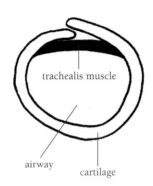

2.5 A cross-sectional view of the trachea showing the incomplete cartilage ring supported by the trachealis muscle.

the cartilage ends and completes the oval structure of the trachea (fig. 2.5). Microscopic hairs called cilia line the trachea and act to filter the air passing into the lungs. The trachea begins to branch upon entering the lungs so that the entire lung area receives a supply of oxygen.

Lungs

The lungs are the area where oxygen is supplied to the blood. This occurs at the end of the airway in little pouches called alveoli. There is a very thin layer of tissue separating the alveoli from the blood vessels. Oxygen easily diffuses from the alveoli, across this tissue layer, and into the blood. Carbon dioxide from the blood diffuses into the alveoli so that it can be expelled during exhalation.

Respiratory Abnormalities

Infectious Respiratory Disease

Miniature horses are susceptible to the same respiratory diseases as full-sized horses, including *influenza, bacterial pneumonia,* and *strangles.* Treatment of these diseases is the same for Miniatures as for large horses, except that medication doses must be appropriately decreased because of their small size.

It is critical that sick Miniature horses are closely monitored for feed intake. Horses frequently go off feed when affected by a respiratory infection. In full-sized horses, this is rarely a problem. In Miniature horses, this can be devastating because of the risk of **hepatic lipidosis** (see Chapter Five). A simple case of influenza (flu) can result in fatal liver failure if the patient goes off feed for several days (or less if the patient is obese).

Caution: Any Miniature horse that has not eaten in 24 hours should be evaluated by a veterinarian to determine if supportive therapy for the liver (forced feeding, intravenous nutrition) should be initiated.

Sinusitis

Sinusitis is a term used to describe infection of a sinus cavity. It may be a primary or secondary disease.

CAUSES

Primary sinusitis is caused by bacteria present in the airway that prolifer-
ate in the sinus. Bacteria gain access to the sinuses from the nasal passageway, especially when bacteria levels are high due to a respiratory
infection.

A risk factor for primary sinusitis in Miniature horses is their relatively
large cheek teeth in relation to the small size of their heads (see Figure 3.1
on p. 48). The teeth fill the sinus, preventing normal sinus drainage and
allowing bacterial proliferation. This is especially a problem in young horses
where the teeth have barely **erupted** into the mouth, leaving a large amount
of root still in the sinus.

Secondary sinusitis is caused by the introduction of bacteria from a source
other than the airway. The most common cause is infection from a tooth root
abscess. Because the wall of bone separating the tooth root from the sinus is
very thin, infection can erode through the bone. In rare cases, the infection
can even spread to other teeth in the sinus.

Any trauma that damages the skin and bone over a sinus leads to contamination of the sinus and the possibility of sinusitis. Even blunt trauma that
does not create a defect can lead to sinusitis if the sinus fills with blood. Blood
acts as a perfect environment for bacterial growth and blood clots can obstruct
the normal drainage of the sinus, further enhancing bacterial proliferation.

A rare cause of secondary sinusitis in horses is a sinus mass, such as a
tumor. The mass can act as a source of infection as well as obstruct normal
sinus drainage.

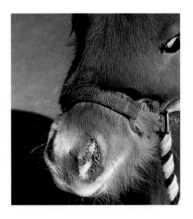

2.6 Classic appearance of
sinusitis—thick, white discharge
from one nostril in an otherwise
healthy horse.

DIAGNOSIS

The most typical sign of sinusitis is **unilateral** nasal discharge (fig. 2.6). The
discharge is usually thick and in some cases will have a foul odor. If the sinus
is unable to drain, the face may swell due to bony remodeling from the
chronic pressure of the built-up fluid. In most cases, the horse will not have
a fever and will show no other signs of illness.

A definitive diagnosis of sinusitis can be made by visualizing fluid in the
sinus with the use of radiographs. Radiographs are also helpful to determine
which sinus is affected and if the infection is secondary to a skull fracture,
tumor, or a tooth root abscess. Placement of an endoscope into the sinus is
a valuable diagnostic tool if radiographs fail to identify an underlying cause
of the sinusitis.

TREATMENT

A mild case of *primary sinusitis* may be treated successfully with antibiotics.
Cases of sinusitis in young horses caused by poor sinus drainage due to

tooth obstruction often respond well to this treatment. This treatment may need to be repeated until the teeth erupt to the point where they no longer occlude the sinus openings.

Cases of primary sinusitis that do not respond to antibiotics require sinus irrigation. A small hole is made in the bone over the sinus. A sample of the pus is collected to identify the type of bacteria causing the infection. Then a tube is placed into the hole so that sterile fluid can be flushed through the sinus. The fluid and infected material then pass out the nose. Repeat treatments are usually necessary. If the outflow tracts of the sinus are completely blocked, a new drainage hole must be created by passing a probe up the nose, and puncturing the thin bone that separates the sinus from the nasal cavity.

In cases of *secondary sinusitis,* the underlying cause must be addressed. In cases of a tooth root abscess, the infected tooth must be removed. This can be done by oral extraction or **repulsion** of the tooth through a hole made in the sinus (see *Dental Extractions,* p. 57).

In cases of trauma, the fracture should be repaired and the skin closed over the defect if possible. If a mass is contributing to the sinusitis, it should be surgically removed. Unfortunately, some tumors are not amenable to surgical resection. The use of radiation therapy may be beneficial in some of these cases.

In all cases of secondary sinusitis, irrigation of the sinus should be performed after the underlying cause has been treated. The use of antibiotics may also be beneficial to resolving the secondary infection.

PROGNOSIS

Most cases of *primary sinusitis* can be resolved with antibiotics and sinus irrigation. The most common complication after treatment of a primary sinusitis is recurrence of the infection. The treatment for repeat cases is the same as for the original infection except that a longer course of antibiotics or more numerous irrigations may be necessary. Surgical exploration of the sinus is recommended if repeat medical therapy fails to resolve the infection.

The prognosis for *secondary sinusitis* depends on the underlying cause. Most cases of traumatic sinusitis can be treated successfully. Benign masses can frequently be removed with good results, but many tumors are difficult or impossible to treat.

The prognosis for secondary sinusitis due to a tooth abscess is guarded to fair. Ongoing infection and the development of communicating tracts between the oral cavity and sinus are common complications. Frequently, multiple surgeries are needed for a successful outcome (see *Dental Extractions,* p. 57).

Choanal Atresia

During the development of the fetus, a membrane is present that separates the nasal passageways from the nasopharynx (fig. 2.7). Early in **gestation,** this membrane ruptures, opening the airway. In rare instances, this membrane fails to rupture and may even ossify (turn to bone). This can occur in one or both nasal passages and is called *choanal atresia.*

DIAGNOSIS

Bilateral *choanal atresia* results in complete airway obstruction due to the obligate nasal respiration of horses. Therefore, foals born with bilateral choanal atresia will be unable to breathe. If emergency treatment is not immediately available, these foals will die in a short period of time.

Unilateral *choanal atresia* is not life threatening and is usually recognized when an owner or trainer realizes that air passes through only one of a horse's nostrils. Passing a scope up the nasal passage will identify the persistent membrane. This also identifies whether the obstruction is a membrane or a bony structure.

TREATMENT

Emergency tracheotomy at birth is indicated in cases of *bilateral choanal atresia.* Surgical correction of the atresia must then be performed as soon as possible. If the membrane has ossified, the skull must be opened to allow access to the obstruction. If the atresia is due to a membrane only, a laser can be passed up the nasal passage and used to cut the membrane. No external incisions are made when laser surgery is performed.

Surgery is an elective procedure in cases of *unilateral choanal atresia.* The correction can be performed at any time, but is most successful after the horse has reached its mature size. If the horse is not making abnormal noise or showing signs of respiratory distress at exercise, surgery is not necessary.

PROGNOSIS

Unfortunately, most foals with *bilateral choanal atresia* die before treatment can be initiated. Many cases of *unilateral atresia* can live comfortable, productive lives without treatment. In those individuals where the atresia interferes with respiration, surgical treatment is often successful. The best results are seen when the atresia is due to an obstructing membrane that can be removed using a laser passed up the nasal passage. More complications are encountered when the skull must be opened to to remove an ossified membrane.

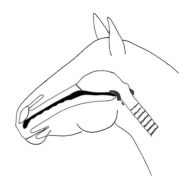

2.7 The red line shows the location of the choanal membrane. During fetal development, two membranes are present, one in each of the nasal passages.

There is a genetic component to this deformity in humans, but the heritability of choanal atresia in horses has not been proven. It is frequently seen in foals with other types of facial and dental malformations and may be associated with dwarfism in Miniature horses (see Chapter Nine). For this reason, removal of any horse with choanal atresia (bilateral or unilateral) from the breeding pool is recommended.

Cleft Palate

Cleft palate is a congenital abnormality where the hard and/or soft palates do not form completely. It is an uncommon defect in all breeds, but has been seen in Miniature horses. While this is not strictly an abnormality of the respiratory system, it frequently leads to pneumonia as feed material passes from the oral cavity, through the cleft palate and into the respiratory tract.

DIAGNOSIS

The most common sign of a cleft palate is milk passing out a foal's nostrils after nursing. The foal may cough while nursing due to milk passing into the trachea. Affected foals frequently develop pneumonia, have little energy and muscle tone, and do not grow normally. The severity of the clinical signs depends on the size of the defect in the palate. Horses with a very small defect have been known to mature normally despite the cleft. A diagnosis of cleft palate in these horses is often made after the animal starts training and is found to have increased respiratory noise or exercise intolerance due to an abnormally functioning soft palate.

A diagnosis of cleft palate in Miniature horses is easily made by examining the back of the mouth with a flashlight. Passing a scope into the oral cavity is recommended to determine the complete extent of the defect.

TREATMENT

Surgical repair is possible. An owner must consider several factors before undertaking this step. First, the surgery is a very painful, invasive procedure. The jaw must be split in order to access the back of the oral cavity. Postoperative complications are common and include infection of the incision or jaw, inability to nurse, failure of the repair, and persistent pneumonia. If the repair is successful, it is unlikely that the horse will be an athletic animal as soft palate dysfunction, which leads to respiratory difficulty at exercise, is frequently a long-term problem.

If the decision to pursue surgery is made, the procedure should be performed as quickly as possible, before the foal develops pneumonia. Any foal that passes milk through its nostrils should be evaluated immediately for a cleft palate.

PROGNOSIS

The prognosis depends on the size and type of cleft palate. If the defect is small and involves only the soft palate, the prognosis for repair is good, but the prognosis for athletic function is guarded because of the possibility of persistent soft palate dysfunction. Multiple surgeries may be needed to complete the repair. Clefts of the hard palate have a poorer prognosis than soft palate defects, and repair of very wide clefts should not be attempted because of the poor prognosis for a successful outcome.

PREVENTION

Because this defect is heritable in humans, a similar genetic predisposition is suspected, but not proven, in horses. Therefore, these animals should not be used for breeding.

Tracheal Collapse

Tracheal collapse occurs when there is a loss of rigidity of the cartilage rings or a flaccidity of the trachealis muscle that bridges them (fig. 2.8). When a horse with a collapsing trachea inhales, the negative pressure causes a flattening of the trachea, resulting in respiratory impairment.

Tracheal collapse can occur in any breed secondary to injury or infection that causes cartilage damage. A primary tracheal collapse syndrome of unknown cause has been seen in Miniature horses and ponies. In other species, primary tracheal collapse has been associated with hereditary or nutritional abnormalities, but this has not been proven in Miniature horses.

DIAGNOSIS

In reported cases of tracheal collapse in Miniature horses, the abnormality occurred only in mature animals. These animals had difficulty breathing whenever stressed or exercised. The degree of respiratory distress experienced by the animal depended on the degree of flaccidity and the length of affected trachea. A diagnosis was made by passing a scope down the trachea and visualizing the collapse.

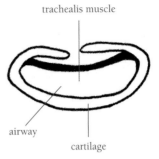

trachealis muscle

airway

cartilage

2.8 A diagram of the cross-sectional area of a collapsing trachea (compare to Figure 2.5). Note that the cartilage does not form a complete ring and the trachealis muscle is thin and flaccid. The airway will narrow even further with the increased force of inhalation that occurs with exercise.

Surgical correction of tracheal collapse is possible in some cases. Surgical approaches that have been used to treat this condition include placement of **prosthesis** around the affected section of trachea to give support to the rings, shortening of the trachealis muscle, and removal of the affected area. None of these surgeries have been consistently successful and complications such as infection and failure of the repair are common.

Tracheal collapse has been shown to have a genetic component in other species. While the heritability of this abnormality in horses has not been proven, owners and breeders should give strong consideration to removing any horse from the breeding pool that develops tracheal collapse with no apparent predisposing cause.

Summary

Miniature horses are susceptible to all of the infectious respiratory diseases that affect other breeds. Sick Miniature horses must be treated aggressively and monitored closely for **anorexia** to prevent hepatic lipidosis.

Sinusitis is a relatively common problem in all horses. Miniature horses are more predisposed to this disease because of the presence of large teeth in their small heads. Owners and veterinarians alike should be suspicious of sinusitis any time a Miniature horse exhibits unilateral nasal discharge. The earlier a diagnosis is reached, the more likely that medical treatment will be successful.

Early treatment is also important for a successful outcome in surgical correction of cleft palate. Any foal that exhibits milk running from its nostril after nursing should be immediately examined for this defect.

Choanal atresia and tracheal collapse are rare in all breeds of horses, but appear to be more common in Miniature horses than in the full-sized horse population. These abnormalities should be considered any time there is evidence of respiratory distress in this breed. Because of the possible heritability of cleft palate, choanal atresia, and tracheal collapse, a horse affected with any of these abnormalities should not be used for reproduction.

CHAPTER 3

The Teeth and Jaws

BECAUSE OF THEIR role in obtaining and processing feed, equine teeth are critical to the survival of the animal. The most common cause of death in aged wild horses is the inability to chew food; these horses either die of intestinal obstruction, weakness, or are taken down by predators.

Dental disease is rarely fatal in domestic horses. Even old horses that have lost most of their teeth can be managed with a soft diet. But healthy teeth are important to the general health of the animal. In addition to affecting the ability of the horse to process its feed, the health of the teeth also affects the health of the sinuses and the condition of the nasal passageway. A normal bite is essential to success in halter classes and a horse must be able to comfortably hold a bit and set its head in order to be successful in driving competitions.

Dental abnormalities such as **malocclusions** and maleruptions are seen more frequently in Miniature horses compared to full-sized animals. This chapter reviews normal dental anatomy, function, and care with emphasis on management of Miniature horses. Dental abnormalities and diseases that are of special concern to Miniature horses will also be addressed.

Normal Dental Anatomy and Maintenance

Structure and Function of the Teeth

The equine tooth is designed to withstand the continuous abrasion of a grass and hay diet. This diet results in the loss of about 0.1 inch (2–3 mm) of tooth surface each year. To compensate for this loss the horse has large teeth that continue to erupt throughout the horse's life, until the tooth is worn to the root. In a young horse, most of the tooth is embedded in the skull or jaw with only a small part of the tooth protruding into the mouth. Wearing of the tooth and loosening of the root is the most common cause of tooth loss in an old horse.

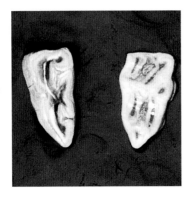

3.1 (above) The comparison of a full-sized horse's tooth to a Miniature horse's tooth. The **occlusal** surface on the left is the right lower second premolar that was removed from a twenty-six-year-old full-sized horse. The occlusal surface on the right is a **cap** removed from the right upper second premolar of a two-year-old Miniature horse.

3.2 (right) The upper dental arcade of a five-year-old stallion. The premolars and molars are referred to as the "cheek" teeth.

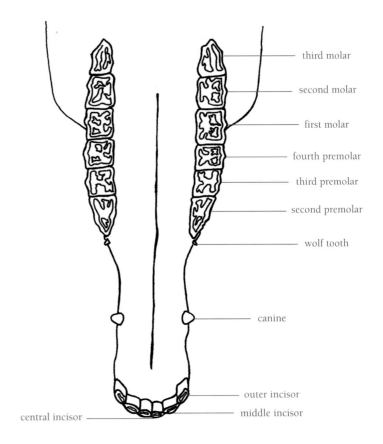

third molar

second molar

first molar

fourth premolar

third premolar

second premolar

wolf tooth

canine

outer incisor

central incisor

middle incisor

Miniature horses have large teeth in relation to their small size (fig. 3.1). Their teeth are only slightly smaller than full-sized horses' teeth. As a result, problems can develop during the development and eruption of the permanent teeth (see **Eruption Bumps,** p. 55 and *Maleruptions,* p. 56).

Dentition

Figure 3.2 shows the dental **arcade** of an adult male horse and Table 1 lists the approximate eruption times of the **deciduous** (temporary) and permanent teeth.

The function of the incisors is to cut grass when the horse is grazing. They play little role in the chewing of food.

The premolars and molars are referred to as the cheek teeth. The function of the cheek teeth is to grind the feed. Their large surface area and their close contact to each other creates the effect of one continuous grinding

TOOTH	DECIDUOUS	PERMANENT
Central Incisor	6 days	2 1/2 years (3 years*)
Middle Incisor	6 weeks	3 1/2 years (4 years*)
Outer Incisor	6 months	4 1/2 years (5 years*)
Canine		4-6 years
Wolf Tooth (First Premolar)	6-18 months	
Second Premolar	Birth to 2 weeks	2 years
Third Premolar	Birth to 2 weeks	3 years
Fourth Premolar	Birth to 2 weeks	4 1/2 years
First Molar		1 year
Second Molar		2 years
Third Molar		3 1/2 years

Table 1 The eruption times of the equine dental arcade. These times can vary with the breed of horse and between individuals. Eruption times marked with an asterisk (*) are those for the mini-Shetland pony population of western Europe.[7] Enough research has not been performed to determine the eruption times for the Miniature horse.

surface on each jaw. The first premolar is a small, nonfunctional tooth called the wolf tooth.

The roots of the last three or four upper cheek teeth are located in the maxillary sinus, an air-filled cavity that lies below the bone in front of each eye. The bone separating the tooth roots from the sinus is thin and easily eroded. Infection of a sinus tooth can easily break through this thin bone, causing a secondary sinus infection (see *Sinusitis,* p. 40).

Dental Wear

Because the lower jaw is narrower than the upper jaw, there is a discrepancy in how the arcades meet, resulting in sharp points along the inside edges of

---

7 Baker GK, Easley J (1999) *Equine Dentistry* WB Saunders, Philadephia, p. 39.

3.3 A A photo of a horse's skull showing how the outside edges of the *upper* teeth do not contact the *lower* teeth. This predisposes to points on the *outside* edges of the upper arcade due to lack of wear (see arrows). Note the presence of a wolf tooth and the absence of canine teeth in this skull (see Figure 3.2).

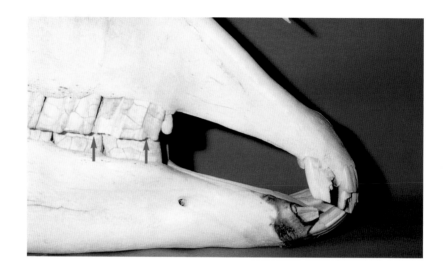

3.3 B The inside of the jaw as viewed from the back of the mouth looking forward. The *inside* edges of the *lower* teeth (seen here) do not contact the *upper* teeth. This predisposes to points on the *lower inside edge* of the arcade due to lack of wear (see arrows).

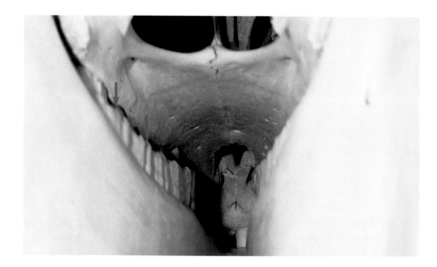

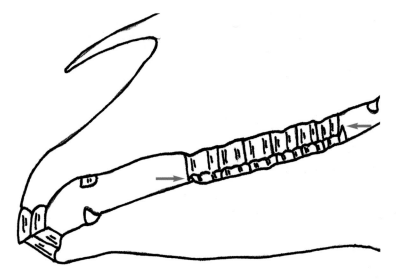

3.4 A normal bite. Because there is a slight overbite of the incisors and cheek teeth, hooks tend to form on the first upper and last lower cheek teeth (see arrows).

the lower teeth and the outside edges of the upper teeth as the teeth wear (figs. 3.3 A & B). Eating or carrying a bit becomes a painful experience for a horse with these points as the sharp edges of the teeth pinch the sensitive inner cheek.

The upper arcade is usually shifted slightly forward of the lower arcade. Consequently, sharp points or **hooks** tend to develop on the upper first cheek teeth and lower last cheek teeth (fig. 3.4). These beak-like over-growths can interfere with the horse's ability to chew, cause discomfort when the horse is bitted, and cause calluses or ulcers on the membranes of the opposite jaw. It is also believed that these hooks can prevent a horse from maintaining a proper headset in harness. When a horse flexes at the poll, the cheek teeth must slide across each other. Hooks prevent this sliding action from taking place and make it uncomfortable for the horse to maintain the flexed position.

Dental Care

Proper dental care begins at birth. The foal's bite and oral cavity should be examined as part of the post-foaling exam. In Miniature horses, oral examinations should then be performed on a monthly basis to check for early signs of malocclusions (dental misalignments) or factors that may predispose to them (see *Sow Mouth*, p. 53). The mouth can also be checked for problems associated with the eruption of the deciduous teeth during these exams. This schedule should be continued through the first six months of life.

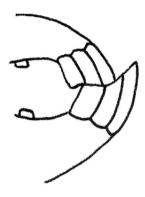

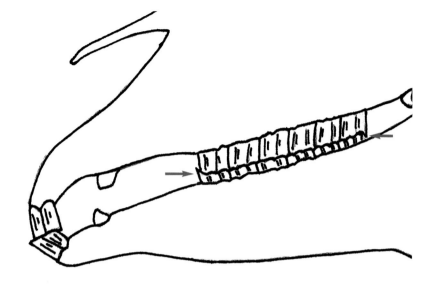

3.5 (above) Sow mouth.

3.6 (right) A sow mouth with affected cheek teeth. Note the hooks forming on the lower first and upper last cheek teeth (see arrows).

After the first six months, the teeth should then be checked twice a year until the horse is four years of age. Dental care during the first four years includes **floating** (filing) of points and hooks, removal of retained remnants of the deciduous teeth, called caps, and correcting problems with erupting teeth.

The wolf teeth will usually erupt in the first year. Because they have no functional significance and may cause irritation from shifting of the tooth or pinching of the cheek against the tooth when a bit is in place, removal of wolf teeth is recommended for any horse that will carry a bit.

A thorough dental exam should be performed before a horse is introduced to a bit. This prevents the development of bad habits associated with the bit that occur because of oral pain.

Once the horse is four years of age, yearly dental exams are usually adequate. However, frequent examinations are necessary if the horse has any dental abnormalities that predispose the teeth to irregular wear. The frequency of examinations may need to be increased as the horse ages. The loss of teeth and the tendency for irregular wear can create problems that make it difficult for the older horse to adequately chew its food.

In addition to routine dental exams, evaluation of the teeth should be performed any time a horse shows signs of dental disease. Indications of possible dental disease include difficulty chewing, dropping of partially chewed food (quidding), excessive salivation, resisting the bit, swelling of the face, nasal discharge, or a foul odor from the mouth or nose.

Malocclusions (Dental Misalignments)

Sow Mouth

Sow mouth (**prognathia**) is a malocclusion where the upper jaw is shorter than the lower jaw (fig. 3.5). This results in the lower incisors projecting in front of the upper incisors. Often, only the incisors are involved, but the deformity may also affect the cheek teeth. This is a relatively common deformity in Miniature horses and while the exact genetics have not been determined, it is considered an inherited abnormality and may be associated with dwarfism (see Chapter Nine).

Because the upper and lower incisors are not in contact with each other, these teeth continue to elongate as they erupt. If left untreated, the upper incisors can lacerate the sensitive tissues behind the lower incisors, and the lower incisors can lacerate the upper gums and lips. In addition, if the cheek teeth are affected, hooks can develop on the lower first cheek teeth and upper last cheek teeth due to incomplete contact between the arcades (fig. 3.6). Horses with a sow mouth need frequent dental care. The incisors must be filed or cut to prevent overgrowth and hooks must be removed.

The eruption of the permanent incisors can give a young Miniature the appearance of a sow mouth. The permanent incisors erupt behind the deciduous teeth, pushing these teeth forward, giving the look of a malocclusion. This is not a true sow mouth, as the horse will have a normal bite as soon as the permanent teeth are in position.

TREATMENT AND PREVENTION

Oral examination of Miniature horse foals that demonstrate a sow mouth has shown that many of these youngsters have an irregularity of the dental arcade called **transverse ridges.** These enamel ridges run across the surface of the upper and lower cheek teeth in a regular, repeating pattern that causes the upper and lower arcade to lock with each other. The effect is of two washboards locked face to face. It is believed that this locking of the premolars and molars inhibits the normal growth of the jaw and predisposes the foal to a sow mouth. Floating to remove these transverse ridges in foals showing the tendency toward a sow mouth will often correct the malocclusion. It is standard practice in many Miniature horse stables for all the youngsters to be checked monthly for transverse ridges and to have these ridges removed before any malocclusion problems develop.

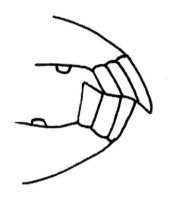

3.7 Parrot mouth.

Another important tool in managing a young horse with a sow mouth is incisor reduction. If the incisors are allowed to become overly long, the upper incisors will lock behind the lower incisors, further inhibiting the growth of the upper jaw. By cutting back the incisors to where they no longer overlap, the malocclusion will often correct itself as the growth of the upper jaw catches up to the lower jaw.

Orthodontic management of this condition is possible in young horses. Ideally, treatment should be initiated no later than three months of age as jaw growth decreases significantly by six months. Treatment consists of application of wires (braces) to the lower jaw that wrap around the incisors and then back around the second premolar. The wires are tightened to inhibit the growth of the lower jaw. The upper jaw continues to grow normally and the deformity is corrected. It is important to remove the wires as soon as correction is obtained to prevent over-correction and the creation of a **parrot mouth.**

Caution: *This procedure should only be undertaken in an attempt to decrease the frequency of dental care and to improve the quality of life for a noncompetitive animal.* The American Miniature Horse Association regulations prohibit the showing of any animal that has had this procedure performed. These horses should not enter the breeding pool, as it is possible for them to pass on this undesirable trait to their offspring.

Parrot Mouth

This is the most common malocclusion in full-sized horses. In a *parrot mouth* (**brachygnathia**), the lower jaw is shorter than the upper jaw, resulting in an overbite (fig. 3.7). The defect is limited to the incisors in some cases and involves the incisors and cheek teeth in others. Like the sow mouth, a parrot mouth prevents normal wear of the incisors and predisposes the horse to formation of hooks. In this case, the lower incisors lacerate the hard palate and hooks form on the first upper cheek teeth and the last lower cheek teeth. Frequent dental care, including incisor reduction, is necessary to manage affected horses.

TREATMENT AND PREVENTION
Transverse ridges and locking of the lower incisors behind the upper incisors may be associated with this malocclusion. Therefore, as in the sow mouth, incisor reduction and floating to remove transverse ridges should be performed. Given time and appropriate dental care, some affected young

horses will grow out of the malocclusion. Orthodontic correction of the deformity is possible with the application of wires to the upper jaw. As with *sow mouth,* the *parrot mouth* affected horse should not be used for breeding and horses that have had wire correction of the defect are not eligible for AMHA competitions.

Dental Abnormalities

Retained Caps

As the deciduous teeth are worn away, the permanent teeth begin to erupt and push the deciduous teeth from their position in the dental arcade. The remnants of the deciduous teeth are called *caps*. In most cases, the caps shed normally and may be found on the ground or in feed tubs. Occasionally, the caps will shift position or become lodged on the permanent tooth. When this occurs, the horse will show evidence of dental discomfort by making abnormal chewing movements, lolling its tongue, or salivating excessively.

TREATMENT
A thorough oral exam should be performed on any horse that is showing signs of oral pain or discomfort. Treatment for horses with dental discomfort associated with retained caps is removal of the caps. In most cases, the horse must be lightly sedated for the procedure. Premature removal of caps should be avoided as it results in exposure of an immature permanent tooth.

Eruption Bumps

Swellings are frequently seen on the head or lower jaw of young Miniature horses. These bumps lie over the tooth roots and are a result of the bone remodeling that occurs during tooth eruptions (fig. 3.8). The bumps are called *teething bumps* or *eruption bumps,* and are a normal physical change that is caused by pressure on the bone from the developing permanent tooth. Eruption bumps are very common in Miniature horses, probably because of the large size of Miniature horse teeth in comparison to the size of their head (see fig. 3.1).

In some cases, the eruption bumps occur internally, in the sinus or nasal cavity. In these cases, the bumps can cause respiratory obstruction. Infection

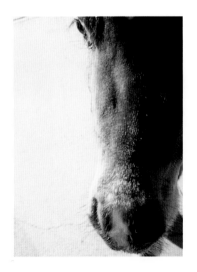

3.8 Eruption bumps on a two-year-old Miniature horse. The swellings on the head below the eye are due to bone remodeling caused by the developing permanent teeth.

of the sinus can also occur when the enlargements block the normal ability of the sinus to drain. These are relatively rare occurrences, but are more frequently seen in Miniature horses than in full-sized horses.

In most cases, eruption bumps resolve as the teeth erupt and the head grows. If the bumps persist or seem to be associated with oral discomfort, the horse should be examined by a veterinarian as this may be an indication of an **impacted** tooth, maleruption (see below), or tooth root abscess. Treatment with antibiotics may be necessary if internal eruption bumps lead to a sinus infection.

Maleruptions and Impactions

Maleruptions and impactions are abnormalities in the normal eruption of the permanent teeth. In maleruptions, the permanent tooth emerges in an abnormal position and in impactions, the permanent tooth is unable to erupt because of insufficient space in the dental arcade. These abnormalities can occur with the incisors or the cheek teeth and are common problems in Miniature horses due to the presence of large teeth in a small head.

Maleruptions of the incisors are most often due to a retained deciduous tooth. The cheek tooth most frequently affected by maleruptions or impactions is the fourth premolar. This is the last cheek tooth to erupt and may become impacted between the third premolar and first molar. When this occurs, swelling develops on the jaw over the affected tooth. The horse may also show signs of oral pain. In some cases, the affected tooth becomes infected.

In rare cases, an impacted upper tooth can erupt inside the arcade through the hard palate. This results in an irregular arcade with a pocket that retains feed material. Retention of the chewed material in the pocket leads to periodontal disease, which could eventually lead to a tooth root abscess.

Because most incisor maleruptions are due to a retained deciduous tooth, extraction of the offending deciduous tooth will eliminate the problem. When the surrounding incisors are too close together to allow eruption of a tooth, their sides can be filed to open up the space.

If a cheek tooth is erupting into its normal position, but becomes lodged between the other teeth, an instrument is inserted between the teeth and used to move them slightly apart to allow room for the impacted tooth to erupt. If a tooth erupts through the hard palate and retention of feed becomes a recurrent problem, the malpositioned tooth should be removed (see *Dental Extractions,* below).

Dental Extractions

An adult tooth must be removed if the tooth is abscessed, fractured, or has erupted in an abnormal position that interferes with the horse's ability to chew or causes pocketing of food material. The cheek teeth are the teeth most commonly affected by these conditions. Because of the length of tooth that is buried in the jaw, the cheek teeth are more difficult to remove than the incisors.

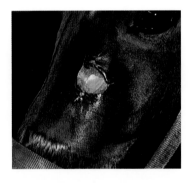

3.9 A Miniature horse with a defect in the skull from repulsion of an upper cheek tooth (second premolar). The defect is packed with gauze.

The affected tooth is removed orally or is pounded out through a hole created in the jaw or sinus, a process called *repulsion.* Oral removal of a tooth in most cases can be performed in a standing, sedated horse. It may take several days to adequately loosen the tooth for removal. The advantages of this procedure are that general anesthesia is avoided and no hole is created in the head as in repulsion. In some cases this cannot be performed. If the affected tooth is very young or barely erupted, it is difficult to get an adequate grip on the tooth to extract it through the mouth. If the tooth or root is badly fractured, all the fragments may not be able to be removed through an oral approach. In these cases, the tooth must be removed by repulsion.

When repulsing a tooth, access to the root of the tooth is gained by creating a hole in the jaw or sinus over the affected tooth. A punch is placed on the root and the tooth is driven out with a hammer. The disadvantages of this procedure include the need for general anesthesia, a higher risk of complications, including fracturing the jaw or injuring a neighboring tooth, and the presence of a defect in the jaw postoperatively, which requires rigorous aftercare (fig. 3.9).

Because of the defect produced in the arcade when a tooth is removed, the opposing tooth will not wear normally. Therefore, frequent dental care is necessary in these animals. Floating twice a year is usually indicated.

In cases of tooth extraction due to an abscess, several complications can be encountered. The most common complications are persistence of the infection in the socket or sinus, spread of the infection to neighboring teeth, and formation of a draining tract between the sinus and the surface of the head where repulsion has been performed. In cases where the tooth was extracted orally, a draining tract can form between the sinus and the oral cavity at the site of tooth removal. Additional surgeries are needed to correct these complications when they occur.

Summary

Miniature horses have a greater tendency to dental problems than full-sized horses with the most commonly seen problems being malocclusions, maleruptions, and impactions. The greater incidence of these abnormalities in Miniature horses is due to the large size of their teeth in relation to their small head. The good news is that most of these problems can be successfully treated if addressed in a timely manner.

CHAPTER 4

Colic

COLIC IS A term used to describe abdominal pain in the horse. It is most commonly seen with gastrointestinal disease, but can also be evidence of urinary tract or reproductive abnormalities. This chapter focuses on **colic** as it relates to the digestive system.

Without a doubt, colic is one of the major health problems faced by horse owners. It is second only to old age as the most common cause of death in all breeds of horses. Miniature horses are at risk for all of the same types of colic seen in full-sized horses, including gas colic, diarrhea, impactions, and twists. However, Miniature horses present unique problems with respect to diagnosing and treating colic. The goal of this chapter is to help Miniature horse owners understand some of the special concerns that come into play when treating their animals for colic.

Anatomy of the Gastrointestinal Tract

Food passes from the mouth, down the esophagus, and into the *stomach.* Acid and digestive enzymes in the stomach begin the digestion process. Swallowed saliva moistens the feed contents and buffers the acid of the stomach. Horses do not vomit. Anatomically, they are capable of vomiting, but the reflex running from the stomach to the brain and back to the stomach that signals the need for vomiting appears to be poorly developed in the horse.

The ingesta (partially digested feed material) then passes into the *small intestine,* which is about 26 feet (7.9 meters) long in the Miniature horse. The functions of the small intestine are to continue the digestion process, absorb fluid and nutrients, and transport the ingesta to the large intestine for further processing.

The first part of the large intestine is the *cecum,* a comma-shaped sac that has a capacity of 1.5–7.0 gallons (5.7–26.5 liters) in the Miniature horse. Microbes present in the cecum digest the fibrous diet of the horse, producing

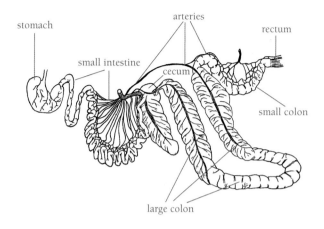

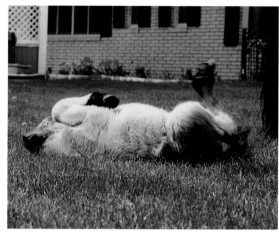

4.1 (above) Anatomy of the equine gastrointestinal tract. The intestines, which have been spread out for clarity, are more closely compacted in the abdomen.

4.2 (above right) Rolling is a common sign of colic in horses.

nutrients essential to the animal. This process is called fermentation and takes about five hours to complete. During this period, a large volume of fluid is absorbed into the body from the feed material.

Ingesta passes from the cecum into the *large colon* where the fermentation process and fluid absorption continue. The large colon measures 3–5 feet (0.9–1.5 meters) in length in Miniature horses. It forms a U-shaped loop that is connected to the body wall only at its beginning and terminal segments. Because of this, the large colon is very mobile within the abdomen, predisposing it to displacements and twists. The diameter of the large colon varies as much as three-fold between adjacent segments. Ingesta can obstruct the more narrow areas, a condition known as impaction.

The processed ingesta then passes into the *small colon*, the final segment of the large intestine. The term *small* colon refers to its small diameter, not its length, which is actually relatively long, measuring about 4 feet (1.2 meters) in Miniature horses. The main function of the small colon is to complete the fluid-absorption process. As fluid is removed from the digested feed, fecal balls are formed and are moved into the *rectum* where they are stored until they are passed from the body (fig. 4.1).

Signs of Colic

The signs of colic vary with the severity of the disease and the horse's tolerance to pain, and may be slow to develop or occur suddenly. The most common signs are the horse looking at its side, pawing, pacing, shaking, sweating, stretching as if to urinate, laying down, and rolling (fig. 4.2). Some horses will spend an excessive amount of time at their water source, playing with, rather than drinking the water. There is often a change in the frequency or consistency of the horse's manure. The horse may develop a bloated appearance due to distension of the intestines with gas or fluid.

In many Miniature horses, the first signs of a serious colic are a depressed attitude and a reluctance to eat, even though they are defecating normally. Other Miniatures in the early stages of colic will continue to eat but will have decreased fecal production with the feces being firmer and drier than normal.

Caution: The possibility of colic should be considered in any Miniature horse that is depressed, off feed, or demonstrating changes in its normal fecal production.

Diagnosing Colic

In most cases, the diagnosis of colic is easily reached based on the horse's pain, decreased gut sounds, and decreased or absent fecal production. The challenge to the veterinarian is to determine the cause of the colic and, therefore, the best treatment approach and the prognosis for survival. Distinguishing between a medical colic and one that requires surgical intervention is critical. This is especially true when the patient must be transported to a surgical facility, miles away. The sooner surgery is performed, the better the chances for a successful outcome.

The Physical Exam

In all cases of colic, the first step in evaluating the patient is the physical exam. The veterinarian uses the physical exam to help determine the horse's degree of pain, hydration status, and bowel activity. Elevated heart and respiratory rates are signs of pain or shock. Dry mucous membranes indicate dehydration. Decreased or absent gut sounds are suggestive of intestinal obstruction and hyperactive gut sounds are an indication of inflammation of the bowel or impending diarrhea.

Nasogastric Intubation

Passage of a *nasogastric* tube is frequently performed as part of the colic examination. The nasogastric tube is a flexible tube that is passed through the nasal passageway, down the esophagus, and into the stomach. A siphon is established to collect fluid from the stomach. A large volume of fluid in the stomach may be an indication of malfunction or blockage of the small intestine. Because horses do not vomit, removal of this excess fluid is critical to prevent rupture of the stomach from fluid overload. The tube also provides a means to administer oral medications such as laxatives.

Abdominocentesis

Abdominocentesis is a procedure where peritoneal fluid is collected from the abdomen. Cells that line the abdomen secrete peritoneal fluid into the abdominal cavity outside of the intestines to lubricate and hydrate the intestines. Changes such as infection, inflammation, or death of the intestine are reflected in the peritoneal fluid. Therefore, collection and analysis of the peritoneal fluid gives the veterinarian an estimate of the health of the bowel.

Rectal Examination

One of the most valuable techniques when determining the cause of colic is the *rectal examination*. The veterinarian palpates the intestines through the wall of the rectum. This is used to evaluate the size and position of the intestines as well as to try and locate an impaction.

Many veterinarians are reluctant to perform a rectal examination in a Miniature horse that is suffering from colic. The small size of the rectum increases the risk of accidentally tearing the rectum during manipulation, a serious and potentially fatal injury. This risk is relatively small in a healthy Miniature horse, but is increased in a colic patient because the patient is often straining from abdominal pain. The risk of a rectal tear is further increased in colic patients that are dehydrated, as the rectum will be very dry and sticky.

Diagnosing the underlying cause of the abdominal pain becomes more difficult if a rectal exam is not performed. Therefore, the veterinarian must make a decision on whether or not to perform a rectal exam based on the risk to the patient and the added information that may be gained from the procedure.

Diagnostic Imaging

Fortunately, the use of *ultrasound examination* and *radiographs,* diagnostics that have limited use in full-sized horses due to the large volume of their abdomen, can be very helpful in evaluating colic in Miniature horses. Much of their abdomen can be visualized with ultrasound and most portable radiograph machines are powerful enough to generate X rays that can penetrate their small abdomen. These diagnostics are used to identify areas of thickened or swollen intestine, assess the degree of intestinal distension (an indication of gas accumulation due to blockage of the bowel), evaluate the positioning of the bowel, and identify impactions or foreign bodies.

Treatment of Colic

In general, the approach to treating colic in Miniature horses is the same as for full-sized animals. Oral and intravenous fluids are used to correct dehydration. Laxatives such as mineral oil are used to lubricate ingesta within the bowel and soften impactions. Dietary modifications are made when needed. For example, complete fasting is often necessary in cases of severe impactions to prevent ingesta from backing-up behind the impaction. Pain relievers, such as nonsteroidal anti-inflammatory drugs (NSAIDs) are used to control the horse's discomfort. Surgery is indicated when the bowel is irreparably damaged or twisted, an obstruction is causing damage to the bowel wall, or the horse is not responding to medical treatment.

Considerations When Treating Miniature Horses for Colic

Hepatic Lipidosis
Of special concern when treating Miniature horses for colic is the risk of *hepatic lipidosis*. Hepatic lipidosis is a type of liver failure that is caused by rapid mobilization of fat stores in a horse that is not eating (see *Hepatic Lipidosis*, p. 82). While this is a rare disease in full-sized horses, Miniatures horses, miniature donkeys, and ponies, especially overweight ones, are prone to this abnormality.

There are several reasons that fasting occurs during colic. Most horses that are experiencing abdominal pain are not interested in eating. Food is often withheld as a form of treatment, especially in cases of impaction colic. Food is also withheld postoperatively to rest the bowel and to allow healing of areas of the intestine that were cut and sutured at surgery. In some patients, the intestines do not function properly after colic surgery and the horse must be fasted until normal bowel activity returns.

All of these situations put a Miniature horse at risk for developing hepatic lipidosis. Therefore, alternate forms of nutrition must be provided. Water can be added to feed pellets and fed in small amounts to minimize stress on a healing bowel. Addition of mineral oil to the slurry may be beneficial during an impaction. In patients where food absolutely must be withheld or the horse is unwilling to eat, intravenous nutrition should be used to prevent rapid fat mobilization.

Nonsteroidal Anti-inflammatory Drugs

Another area where care must be taken when managing a Miniature horse with colic is the use of pain relievers. The most commonly used pain relievers are the NSAIDs *phenylbutazone* and *flunixin meglumine* (Banamine®). These drugs not only minimize the horse's discomfort, they also may help to normalize the activity of the bowel, making them valuable tools in the treatment of colic. However, they must be used with caution. The horse's level of pain is an important indicator of the seriousness of the colic. Continued discomfort despite medical treatment is an indication that surgery should be considered. Inappropriate use of NSAIDs will mask the signs of pain, delaying surgery to the point where a successful outcome is unlikely. Administration of NSAIDs before the veterinarian has examined the horse can make an accurate diagnosis of the underlying cause of the colic even more difficult.

These concerns about the use of NSAIDs hold true for all horses, but are even more of a worry in Miniature horses. In full-sized horses, repeat rectal examinations are used to follow the course of the colic and the horse's response to treatment. Multiple rectal examinations can be a risky procedure and are often not performed in Miniature horses. Instead, veterinarians rely more on the horse's level of pain as an indicator of the progression of the colic. Also, because of their small size and the difficulty estimating their weight, NSAIDs can easily be overdosed in Miniature horses (see *Laminitis Treatment*, p. 12, for the appropriate dosing of NSAIDs). Not only does this mask the gravity of the colic, it puts the animal at risk for kidney failure and ulceration of the stomach and colon (see fig. 1.13). The risk of kidney failure is further increased when overdoses occur in a horse that is not drinking adequate amounts of water. For these reasons, NSAIDs should be used to treat colic patients only under the supervision of a veterinarian.

Adhesions

An adhesion is scar tissue that forms in the abdomen (fig. 4.3). Any type of inflammation or infection in the abdominal cavity can lead to adhesion formation. The most common cause of intra-abdominal inflammation and infection is damage to the bowel from a twist or obstruction. The greater the degree of damage, the greater is the risk of adhesions.

Adhesions can cause obstruction of the bowel by impinging on its diameter or twisting around it like a tie. When the adhesion completely

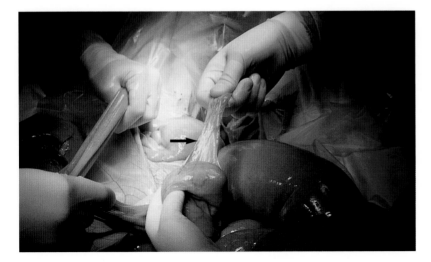

4.3 An adhesion to the small intestine (arrow). This adhesion caused an **acute** colic episode as it twisted around the small intestine, cutting off the flow of ingesta through the bowel.

obstructs the bowel, the horse experiences a severe colic episode. Partial obstruction of the bowel by an adhesion usually results in low-grade, repeat colic episodes due to impactions forming at the narrowed area of the bowel.

All horses are at risk for adhesions, but Miniature horses form adhesions to a greater extent than full-sized horses do. When treatment of colic is delayed, or immediate surgery is not performed when indicated, Miniature horses are placed at risk for future colic problems due to adhesions. Prompt treatment of colic minimizes injury to the bowel and improves the prognosis for a successful long-term outcome.

When to Call the Veterinarian

A common question from horse owners is "When do I call the vet when my horse is colicking?" Many owners opt to call their veterinarian at the first signs of abdominal pain. This is, without a doubt, the safest approach. Other owners prefer to wait-and-see. As some episodes of colic can resolve without treatment, this is a reasonable strategy, as long as the horse is being closely monitored for worsening of the colic.

The following are general guidelines for when it is time to seek veterinary care for a colicky horse.

- The horse has been walked or longed for over an hour and it is still in pain.
- The horse is unwilling to stay on its feet.

- The horse is rolling.
- The horse is not apparently in pain, but has not eaten or defecated for six hours.

Common Causes of Colic in Miniature Horses

Gas and Spasmodic Colic

CAUSES

Gas and *spasmodic colic* are the most common types of colic in all horses. In most cases, the cause of the colic cannot be determined, but parasite infestation, inappropriate feeding habits, rapid changes in feed, or feeding overly rich or poor-quality hay may induce a gas or spasmodic colic.

DIAGNOSIS

Signs of *gas colic* include pain, decreased or absent gut sounds, and gas distension of the bowel that can be palpated on rectal examination or visualized on radiographs. The horse can be in a lot of pain if the gas distension is severe. Usually, the horse is not defecating.

Signs of *spasmodic colic* include pain and hyperactive gut sounds. The movements of the bowel are not coordinated enough to move the ingesta through the intestines. Therefore, affected horses do not defecate despite the apparent activity of the bowel.

TREATMENT

Treatment for gas and spasmodic colic consists of correcting dehydration or electrolyte imbalances and providing pain relief. Exercising the horse on a longe line will often stimulate the bowel to pass the gas or return to a more normal motility pattern

Close monitoring of a horse being treated for gas or spasmodic colic is critical. These types of colic can appear very similar to early intestinal twists and displacements. If a horse continues to be distended and in pain despite treatment, a twist may be present and surgical exploration of the abdomen is indicated. Excessive use of pain relievers could mask ongoing signs of pain, causing a dangerous delay in surgery.

PROGNOSIS

Most patients with gas and spasmodic colic respond well to treatment. The exception is those cases that progress to a twisted or displaced colon due to the changes in motility that occur with these types of colic. It is impossible to predict which cases will develop a large colon twist or displacement; therefore, all cases of gas and spasmodic colic should be monitored closely for continuing or worsening pain.

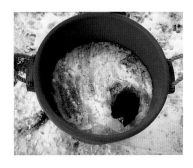

4.4 This photo of a water tub was taken by the author at a farm where two horses were treated for colic on the same day. It is not surprising that the horses were not drinking adequate amounts of water.

PREVENTION

While many gas and spasmodic colics cannot be prevented, good management techniques go a long way toward minimizing the incidence of these diseases. Horses should have regular deworming and dental care. Feeding multiple, small meals of good quality feed is recommended. The bulk of horses' diets should consist of forage (grass, hay, beet pulp) with only a small percentage of the daily calories provided by grain. Horses should have access to clean, fresh, unfrozen water at all times (fig. 4.4) and all changes in feed should be made gradually. A study on feeding practices associated with colic showed that a change in the batch of hay or type of grain or concentrate increases the risk of colic in horses.[8]

Impaction

Impaction, a blockage in the intestine caused by ingested material, is another relatively common cause of colic in horses. Common sites of impactions are the stomach, cecum, large colon (especially where the diameter narrows), and the small colon.

CAUSES

Most impactions consist of coarse, dry-feed material (see below), but can also be caused by foreign bodies, concretions of plant material and hair, ascarids (roundworms) or sand (see *Sand Colic,* p. 70). Persimmon seed ingestion is a frequent cause of stomach impactions in regions where persimmons are grown. Ascarid impactions most typically occur after deworming a young horse with a heavy worm infestation. The dead worms form an obstruction that is most commonly seen in the small intestine. **Fecaliths** and **enteroliths** are special types of impactions and will be discussed individually (see pp. 74 and 76).

Impactions consisting of dry-feed material may be caused by inadequate water intake, poor chewing of feed because of dental disease, or a decrease in physical activity that can affect the bowel motility. Impactions are fairly common in old horses, probably because of tooth loss and age-related decreased motility of the colon.

8 Hudson JM, Cohen ND, Gibbs PG, Thompson JA. Feeding practices associated with colic in horses. *J Am Vet Med Assoc* 2001; 219: 1419

Signs of an impaction include loss of appetite, decreased-to-absent gut sounds, and decreased fecal production. The degree of pain varies from mild discomfort to severe, unrelenting pain, depending on the size of the impaction and the degree of distension (stretching) of the bowel associated with it.

While most large intestinal impactions in full-sized horses can be palpated rectally, as I mentioned earlier, many veterinarians elect to not perform a rectal examination in Miniature horses when they are suspicious of an impaction. As most horses with impactions have some degree of dehydration, there is an increased risk of rectal tearing in these cases. The impaction may be visible on radiographs, making this a good alternative to rectal examination in Miniature horses.

TREATMENT

Treatment consists of softening the impaction with laxatives and fluids, and providing pain relief. Laxatives are either lubricants such as mineral oil, or irritants, such as Epsom salts, that draw fluid into the intestine. They are administered through a nasogastric tube. Fluids are given either through a nasogastric tube, intravenously, or injected into the impaction at surgery.

Pain relief is usually provided by the use of NSAIDs. As mentioned in the section on treatment of colic, caution must be exercised when using these medications. The horse's level of comfort is a key indicator of response to treatment. Excessive use of pain relievers gives the horse the appearance of improvement, even when the impaction and health of the bowel are worsening. Discomfort may not become evident until the impaction has progressed to the point where treatment is unlikely to be successful. This is a special concern in Miniature horses where repeat rectal exams to evaluate the size and softness of the impaction are not practical. It is important to remember that the use of pain relievers will make the horse feel better, and therefore want to eat, even when the impaction is still present. Care must be taken not to overfeed a horse with an impaction that is on NSAIDs as this may lead to an increase in the size of the blockage.

In full-sized horses, feed is withheld until the impaction is almost cleared. Again, this should be done with caution in Miniature horses because of the risk of hepatic lipidosis (see *Hepatic Lipidosis*, p. 82.) Instead, the feed should be changed to a low volume, laxative feed. Small amounts of complete-feed slurry with mineral oil is one alternative to fasting. In severe impactions where food must be withheld, intravenous nutrition should be provided to protect the liver.

How well the horse responds to treatment depends on the extent of the impaction. Treatment with a single-dose laxative is often enough to resolve the obstruction. In other cases, intravenous fluids and multiple laxative doses are necessary. If the impaction is not resolving, the horse remains in pain despite medication, or fluid collected from the abdomen shows damage to the bowel from the weight and pressure of the impaction, surgical intervention is necessary.

There are two approaches to relieving impactions surgically. First, fluid can be injected directly into the impaction followed by massage to break up the mass. If the impaction is very hard or large, the bowel must be opened to remove the obstruction.

The most common complications after surgical treatment of impactions in Miniature horses are adhesion formation (especially if the bowel was damaged or inflamed from the impaction), infection (a greater risk if the bowel was opened to relieve the impaction), and hepatic lipidosis if the horse is unwilling to eat postoperatively.

After the impaction has been relieved, feed is gradually introduced to the horse. The horse must be closely monitored for several days for signs of recurrence of the impaction. Signs that another impaction may be forming include decreased fecal production, decreased or absent gut sounds, and colic.

PROGNOSIS

The prognosis for impactions depends of the severity of the obstruction. If the impaction is not overly dry or large and the bowel is still healthy, there is a good chance that the impaction will resolve with oral fluids and laxatives. Larger, firmer obstructions may require the use of intravenous fluids to soften the impaction, but as long as the horse remains comfortable and abdominocentesis (see p. 62) shows that the bowel has not been damaged, there is still a good chance that the impaction can be resolved without surgery.

The prognosis becomes significantly poorer if surgery is required. This is because surgery is performed only on the most severe impactions that have not responded to medical treatment. Frequently the bowel is already damaged, increasing the risk for postoperative peritonitis and adhesion formation, as well as rupture of the bowel during surgical manipulations. One study showed a 95 percent long-term survival rate after medical treatment of impactions.[9] The survival rate decreased to 58 percent in horses that required surgical intervention.

9 Dabareiner RM, White NA. Large colon impaction in horses: 147 cases (1985-1991). *J Am Vet Med Assoc*1995; 206: 679

Impactions are one of the most preventable types of colic. Regular dental care, free-choice access to fresh, clean, non-frozen water (fig. 4.4), and use of only good quality feed are important preventive steps. Horses should have regular exercise or access to turnout. Proper deworming of pregnant mares and early initiation of a deworming program in foals will prevent ascarid impactions. Prevention of sand impactions is discussed in the next section.

Owners should be familiar with their horses' normal fecal production as the earliest sign of an impaction is abnormally firm feces or decreased fecal production. This is especially true in old horses and horses that must be confined to a stall (such as after an injury). Early, aggressive treatment gives the best chance for a successful outcome.

Sand Colitis and Impaction

CAUSE

Horses that are housed in a sandy environment are at risk for *sand* **colitis** (inflammation of the large intestine) and *impactions*. The horse picks up bits of sand in the process of finishing its feed. As most Miniature horses are on restricted diets because of their tendency to become overweight, they tend to ingest sand when trying to clean up every last morsel of food. Foals will sometimes develop the habit of eating sand and dirt. The cause for this is unknown and may go on for several months before the foal stops this undesirable behavior.

Because of its weight, the sand settles out in the bowel instead of passing through with the rest of the fecal material. Sand is very irritating to the bowel wall, resulting in pain and decreased absorption of nutrients. If the horse's water intake is decreased or large volumes of sand accumulate, a sand impaction may develop.

DIAGNOSIS

Signs of sand colitis are decreased appetite, weight loss, diarrhea, and colic. Gut sounds may be decreased or increased. Depending of the severity of the colitis, the horse may be dehydrated, or showing signs of shock. Sand can often be heard moving in the bowel sitting at the bottom of the abdomen, producing a sound like waves washing over a beach. Sand may be seen in the feces, but the lack of sand in the fecal material does not rule out the presence of sand in the bowel. Radiographs are very useful in identifying the presence of sand throughout the gastrointestinal tract (fig. 4.5).

The horse usually experiences more pain with a sand impaction than with sand colitis. The pain is due not only to distension of bowel in front of the

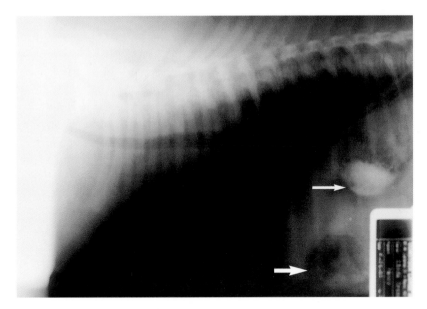

4.5 This radiograph was taken to check for pneumonia in a three-week-old foal (the black area is air-filled lungs). An additional finding was a large amount of sand in the stomach (see small arrow) and the large colon (large arrow).

impaction, but also due to the weight of the sand on the intestines. Passing of small volumes of liquid, sandy feces is very suggestive of a sand impaction. If the impaction has caused damage to the bowel, the horse may show signs of shock. Again, radiographs can be used for a definitive diagnosis.

TREATMENT

The first step in treatment of sand colitis or impaction is to remove the patient from the sandy environment. In mild cases, this may be all that is needed to give the horse a chance to pass the sand. In more severe cases, intravenous fluids are needed to correct dehydration, address electrolyte abnormalities, treat shock, and hydrate the impaction. Laxatives are beneficial for softening the impaction. If there are signs that the bowel is damaged, antibiotics are recommended.

The veterinarian may use psyllium to treat sand colitis and impactions. Psyllium is a fiber supplement that binds the sand and helps move it through the bowel. One study showed no benefit to its use, but many veterinarians have used it successfully.[10] It is initially administered through a nasogastric tube, but once the horse is eating well, it can be mixed with feed.

Occasionally, a sand impaction does not respond to medical treatment and surgical removal of the sand is required (fig. 4.6). Unfortunately, by the time surgery is performed, the bowel is often severely damaged. This weakening of the bowel and the weight of the sand increases the chance of rupture of the

10 Hammock PD, Freeman DE, Baker GJ. Failure of psyllium mucilloid to hasten evacuation of sand from the equine large intestine. *Vet Surg* 1998; 27: 547

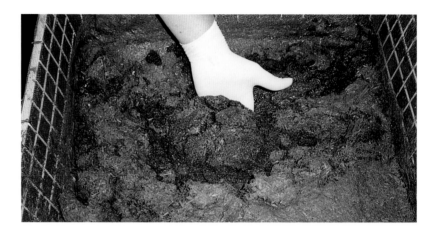

4.6 Material removed from the large colon of a Miniature horse at surgery. On first glance, it appeared to be fecal material. Closer examination revealed it to be sand and gravel coated with ingesta. This Miniature horse weighed 195 pounds (88.6 kg) before surgery. Thirty-two pounds (14.5 kg) of sand were removed from her colon.

bowel during surgical manipulation. The inflammation of the bowel also increases the chance of postoperative infection and adhesion formation.

PROGNOSIS

The prognosis for mild cases of sand colic is good. Most of these horses respond well to removal from the sandy environment, oral laxatives, and oral or intravenous fluids. However, if there is evidence that the bowel is damaged (abnormal fluid obtained on abdominocentesis, or signs of shock in the patient) the prognosis is much poorer.

The prognosis also decreases in horses requiring surgery for sand impaction. Frequently, the bowel is already severely damaged by the time surgery is preformed. The survival rate for horses having surgery for sand impactions is only about 60 percent.[11] Early surgical intervention gives the best chance for postoperative survival.

PREVENTION

Several steps can be taken to decrease the risk of sand colitis and impaction. The most important is to minimize the horse's exposure to sand. Mats can be placed in the area where the horse is fed to decrease ingestion of sand with the feed. Horses that are fed in feeders are not protected from sand ingestion as horses will pull their feed out of the feeder and eat it off the ground.

Foals that have developed the habit of eating dirt and sand must be kept completely off these surfaces. Their stalls and paddocks must be covered in mats or carpet. Placing bedding over a sand surface is not adequate, as the foals will dig through the bedding to get to the sand beneath. Pasture turnout is sometimes beneficial for these youngsters, but they should be

11 Ragle CA, Meagher DM, Lacroix CA, Honnas CM. Surgical treatment of sand colic. Results in 40 horses. *Vet Surg* 1989; 18: 48

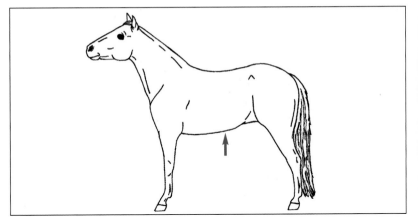

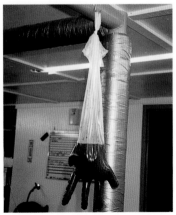

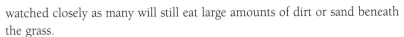

watched closely as many will still eat large amounts of dirt or sand beneath the grass.

Periodic administration of psyllium may be helpful in clearing small amounts of sand from the large colon and is recommended for any horse being fed in a sandy area. The psyllium should be fed once or twice a week, or for several days in a row, once or twice a month. Daily feeding may interfere with the horse's absorption of nutrients and decrease the effectiveness of the psyllium. The best approach is to consult with the horse's veterinarian to determine the most appropriate psyllium-feeding schedule.

It is important for owners of horses that are at risk for sand ingestion to learn to monitor the horse for sand. The first method is to listen for sand in the bowel. To do this, a stethoscope is placed at the lowest point of the abdomen and the gut sounds monitored for one to two minutes (fig. 4.7). Any "beach" sounds are indicative of the presence of sand.

Another test for sand is to perform a fecal sand test. A handful of fresh feces are collected and placed in a plastic bag. It is important that dirt or sand is not picked up off the ground with the feces. The feces are mixed with water and the bag hung for five to ten minutes (fig. 4.8). If the horse has been ingesting sand, it will settle out in the bottom of the bag. Even a small amount of sand can be identified by feeling through the plastic bag.

These tests do not give any information about the health of the bowel or the amount of sand present in it. But a positive test does indicate that management changes must be made to prevent further sand ingestion. If any of these tests are positive and the horse is showing any other signs of sand colitis or impaction, a veterinarian should be contacted immediately so that treatment can be initiated.

Perhaps the most accurate method of determining if sand is present in the bowel is to radiograph the abdomen. This is especially useful in Miniature

4.7 (left) To listen for "beach" sounds to diagnose sand in the colon, place the stethoscope at the lowest point of the abdomen.

4.8 (above) A fecal float for sand. The tips of the rectal sleeve are carefully palpated for sand. A plastic bag can also be used.

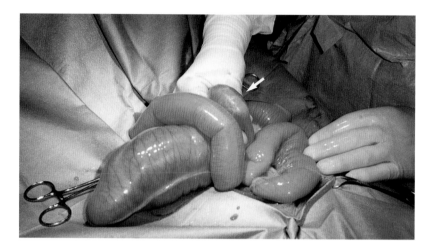

4.9 A fecalith in the small colon of a Miniature horse (see arrow). Notice that the color has blanched from the intestine at the site of the fecalith. This is an indication of decreased blood flow to the bowel caused by the pressure of the obstruction.

horses because their small size results in very clear radiographs of the abdomen, which not only allow the veterinarian to identify the presence of sand, but also helps in estimating the amount of sand that is present and which section of the intestines is most affected (see fig. 4.5).

Fecaliths

Fecaliths are a specific type of impaction that occurs in the small colon (fig. 4.9). They are seen in all breeds of horses, but are much more common in Miniatures, being the most common cause of colic in Miniature horses. Any age horse can be affected, but younger horses are at greater risk of fecalith formation. Common age groups are sucklings and weanlings that are being introduced to a more solid feed.

CAUSE
Fecaliths are composed of dry, fibrous fecal material and are believed to be a result of improper fecal-ball formation. Other materials such as hair, sand, or foreign bodies may be associated with the fecal material (fig. 4.10). Because fecaliths are larger and dryer than normal fecal balls, they become stuck in the small colon.

DIAGNOSIS
The two most common signs of a fecalith are colic and a stop in fecal production. The degree of pain depends on the amount of distension of the bowel in front of the fecalith. In some cases, the horse will develop a bloated appearance due to gas distension of the colon. Gut sounds are decreased or

absent in most cases, but may be increased in the early stages of the obstruction as the body tries to pass the obstruction.

The best way to definitively diagnose a fecalith is by the use of contrast radiography. An enema is performed using a liquid contrast material that is especially designed to show up on radiographs. The location of the fecalith is then identified as the area where the contrast material stops in its movement up the bowel (fig. 4.11). This procedure is best performed in a heavily sedated or anesthetized horse, as an awake animal will repeatedly strain to pass the contrast material.

TREATMENT

Treatment of fecaliths is the same as for other types of impactions. Fecaliths tend to have a poorer response to medical treatment than large-colon impactions. Horses also tend to be in more pain with fecaliths as the entire large colon becomes distended with gas due to the blockage in the small colon. For these reasons, surgical intervention is more common with fecaliths than with other types of impactions.

The decision for surgery should not be overly delayed in Miniature horses. Usually the horse is unwilling to eat, which increases the risk of hepatic lipidosis. Also, the pressure of the fecalith on the wall of the bowel causes inflammation that can lead to postoperative adhesions. A general guideline is that surgery should be considered if the horse has not passed the impaction after 24 hours of aggressive medical treatment (intravenous fluids, laxatives). Surgical intervention should be performed immediately if fluid collected from the abdomen shows evidence of degeneration of the bowel wall, or if the horse develops unrelenting pain. Again, pain relievers should be used with caution so that signs of deterioration are not masked.

PROGNOSIS

The prognosis for survival in Miniature horses that have surgery for treatment of fecaliths is fair. The most common complication is recurrence of the blockage. This may occur as soon as one to two days postoperatively in some patients. These horses may have abnormal small-colon motility that predisposes them to this problem. In general, if immediate re-obstruction does not occur, the prognosis for long-term survival improves significantly.

PREVENTION

Steps to prevent fecaliths are the same as for other types of impactions. In addition, Miniature horses should be fed only high-quality immature forages. As fecaliths are more common in young Miniature horses, low-bulk diets are recommended until the foal is at least six months of age. As hair

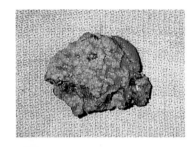

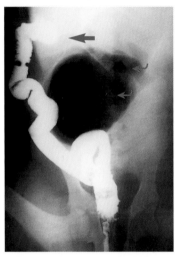

4.10 (top) The fecalith pictured in Figure 4.9 after removal from the intestine. This fecalith was made up of sand, hair, and feces.

4.11 (bottom) A contrast radiograph to identify obstruction by a fecalith. A catheter is placed in the rectum (small arrow) and the liquid contrast (shown as white on the radiograph) is injected. The forward movement of the contrast stops at the location of the fecalith (large arrow). The large black area in the center of the radiograph (curved arrows) is gas in the large colon that has accumulated due to the obstruction.

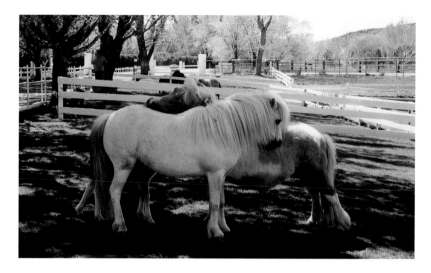

4.12 Mutual grooming may lead to the formation of fecaliths, especially during shedding season.

is a relatively common component of fecaliths, aggressive grooming or even body clipping in the spring may help prevent fecalith formation around hair balls that form during mutual grooming activities (fig. 4.12).

To help prevent recurrence of fecaliths, horses should be fed a low-bulk diet for at least several weeks after treatment. Complete feed pellets or access to pasture are good choices for management. Horses that have had more than one fecalith should be kept on this diet for life.

Enteroliths

Enteroliths are stone-like concretions that can obstruct the large or small colon. A study performed in Texas on the risk factors associated with the development of enteroliths showed that of all breeds of horses, Arabians and Miniature horses are at the highest risk for enterolith formation.[12]

CAUSE

Enteroliths are primarily composed of ammonium magnesium phosphate that is deposited in layers around a foreign body such as metal, wood, or even hair. Enteroliths form in a variety of shapes and sizes (fig. 4.13).

Ammonia is produced in the large colon, phosphate is present in feed, and the magnesium is ingested in feed and water. Magnesium levels in feed and water vary in different areas of the country. Therefore, the occurrence of enteroliths also varies from region to region.

12 Ragle CA, Meagher DM, Lacroix CA, Honnas CM. Surgical treatment of sand colic. Results in 40 horses. *Vet Surg* 1989; 18: 48

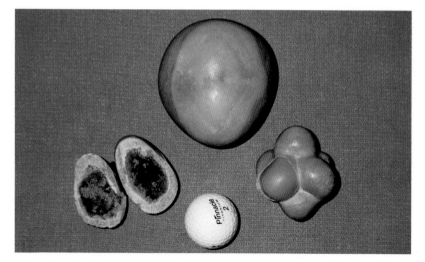

4.13 Various enteroliths that have been removed from Miniature horses. One has been split to show an accumulation of hair that acted as the nidus (point of origin) for formation of the stone. The golf ball is included for size comparison.

DIAGNOSIS

Signs of an enterolith vary depending on its size and location. No signs may be seen with a small stone; apparently normal horses have been known to pass stones in their feces. Larger enteroliths may cause irritability, decreased performance, and intermittent colic. Clinical signs typical of an impaction occur when the enterolith causes complete obstruction of the bowel. Horses may be in severe pain if the bowel in front of the enterolith becomes distended. Signs of shock may develop if the bowel wall is damaged.

A veterinarian will become suspicious of an enterolith if the horse is showing signs of colic and has ceased to pass feces. Chronic, recurrent colic is also suggestive of the presence of an enterolith. This suspicion will be greater if the horse is from an area of the country where enteroliths are common. Enteroliths can be seen on radiographs, making this a valuable diagnostic tool (fig. 4.14).

TREATMENT

Treatment is surgical removal of the enterolith. The best chance for a successful surgery and recovery is if the surgery is performed before the bowel becomes damaged. This decreases the chance of infection and adhesions, and eliminates the need to remove injured bowel.

PROGNOSIS

The prognosis for recovery from surgery to remove an enterolith is excellent. One study showed a 96 percent long-term survival rate postoperatively with recurrence of an enterolith in only 7.7 percent of the patients.[13]

---

13 Hassel DM, Langer DL, Snyder JR, Drake CM, Goodell ML, Wyle A. Evaluation of enterolithiasis in equids: 900 cases (1973-1996). *J Am Vet Med Assoc* 1999; 214: 233

4.14 A radiograph of a horse's abdomen, showing the presence of an enterolith (see large arrow) in the large colon, directly behind the liver (small arrow).

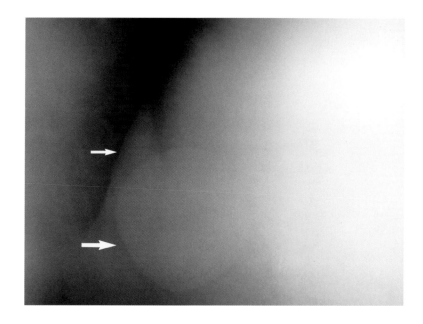

PREVENTION
Studies have been performed to determine the risk factors for formation of enteroliths (see Footnotes [12] and [13]). Feeding alfalfa hay and keeping a horse confined more than 50% of the time are two risk factors identified in the studies. The minerals in the alfalfa may predispose the horse to enterolith formation and confinement may alter normal intestinal activity, thereby providing an opportunity for the stone to form. Minimizing confinement and eliminating alfalfa hay from the diet of Miniature horses is recommended, especially in those areas of the country where enteroliths are common. Owners should consult with their veterinarian to determine if they are in a high-risk area.

Summary

Colic is a common disease in all breeds of horses. However, because of the risk of *hepatic lipidosis* and the increased tendency for adhesion formation, early, aggressive treatment of colic in Miniature horses is even more critical than in full-sized animals. Fortunately, in most cases that are treated in a timely manner, Miniature horses recover well from medical and surgical colic.

CHAPTER 5

The Liver, Hyperlipemia,
and Hepatic Lipidosis

A HEALTHY LIVER is vital to the survival of any animal. While liver diseases are infrequently seen in horses, hepatic lipidosis, a rare problem in full-sized horses, is a common cause of liver failure in Miniatures. An understanding of liver function is critical to the understanding of this disease and its precursor, **hyperlipemia.**

Normal Liver Function

The liver performs several functions critical to an animal's survival. It produces and secretes bile that is important in digestion. It acts as the filtering system of the blood returning from the intestines, removing toxins and infectious organisms before they have a chance to enter the general circulation. One of the most important roles of the liver is the maintenance of energy sources for the body.

Fatty acids and amino acids are created during digestion and fermentation of feed. The fatty acids and amino acids are absorbed into the bloodstream and transported to the liver where they are used to manufacture glucose. Glucose is used to meet the immediate energy demands of the horse and excess glucose is converted to glycogen, which is stored in the liver and muscle for future energy needs (fig. 5.1).

When glucose and glycogen energy stores are depleted, such as during periods of fasting or stress, fatty acids, absorbed from the intestines and mobilized from fat stores, become the primary energy source. If the delivery of fatty acids to the liver overwhelms the liver's ability to process them, the fat is stored in the liver (fig. 5.2).

Hyperlipemia

Hyperlipemia is the term used to describe excess fat products, including triglycerides, cholesterol, and fatty acids, in the blood. It is a result of

5.1 The normal processing of energy sources by the liver.

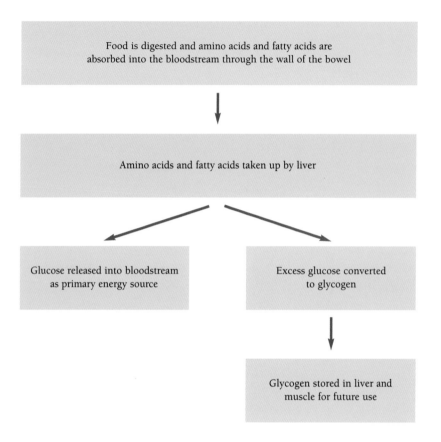

Food is digested and amino acids and fatty acids are absorbed into the bloodstream through the wall of the bowel

Amino acids and fatty acids taken up by liver

Glucose released into bloodstream as primary energy source

Excess glucose converted to glycogen

Glycogen stored in liver and muscle for future use

rapid fat metabolism during times of decreased feed intake or increased energy demands due to stress. Fat mobilization is more rapid than liver uptake, causing increased levels of fat in the blood.

CAUSE

Anorexia due to the presence of another primary disease, such as colic or respiratory infection, is a frequent cause of hyperlipemia. Increased stress, such as what occurs during transportation, late gestation, early lactation, or weaning can also initiate the disease. The likelihood that a horse will develop hyperlipemia is greatest in overweight animals where fat mobilization is quite rapid. Horses affected with *Cushing's disease* (see p. 85) are at greater risk for hyperlipemia than a normal horse.

DIAGNOSIS

Miniature horses, ponies, and miniature donkeys are at greater risk for hyperlipemia than full-sized horses. Therefore, the possibility of hyperlipemia

5.2 Processing of energy stores during hyperlipemia and hepatic lipidosis.

should be considered in any Miniature horse that is off feed. The anorexia may be the initiating cause, or may be the result of the loss of appetite that occurs during hyperlipemia. Other clinical signs of hyperlipemia include diarrhea, weakness, and depression.

Hyperlipemia can be seen in blood drawn for analysis. The fat products will cause the blood and **serum** to have a whitish discoloration. Measuring the levels of triglycerides in the blood gives a quantitative measure of the degree of hyperlipemia.

TREATMENT

Caution: Immediate treatment should be initiated in any animal suspected of having hyperlipemia to prevent progression of the disease to hepatic lipidosis (see below). Intake of carbohydrate-rich feed, such as molasses-coated grain and high quality pasture or hay, should be encouraged. If the horse will not eat, or the hyperlipemia is severe, intravenous nutrition (dextrose) should be administered. Bloodwork should be performed to monitor the liver closely for hepatic lipidosis.

The primary disease or stress must be addressed. Aggressive treatment of medical disorders such as colic or infection is critical to decrease the strain on the body and improve the animal's appetite. If hyperlipemia develops during transport, the animal should be removed from the transport vehicle and allowed to recover before further hauling takes place. Induction of labor may be necessary in late-term mares affected by hyperlipemia. The foal should then be raised as an orphan in order to prevent further demands on the mare. Foals should also be removed from lactating mares that develop hyperlipemia. The best approach is to place the foal where the mare can see and touch it, but it cannot nurse. This prevents aggravation of the disease from the stress of weaning. All foals should be weaned with as little trauma as possible to protect the foal and the mare from this disease.

Hepatic Lipidosis

Uncontrolled hyperlipemia leads to *hepatic lipidosis* (fatty liver disease). The liver takes up the fat from the blood. When the processing of the fat cannot keep up with the amount of fat that is delivered, the fat is stored throughout the tissue of the liver. The fat infiltration interferes with normal liver function leading to failure or rupture of the liver.

DIAGNOSIS

The signs are the same as for hyperlipemia with the addition of symptoms caused by liver dysfunction and liver failure. Mild colic, jaundice, fever, and fluid swelling of the lower abdomen and legs frequently occur. In the most severe cases, changes in mental awareness ranging from mild confusion to uncontrolled behavior and coma may develop due to metabolic toxins that are normally processed and eliminated in the liver reaching the brain. Blood work can be used to diagnose hepatic lipidosis by the presence of hyperlipemia and elevated liver enzymes.

TREATMENT

Treatment of hepatic lipidosis is the same as for hyperlipemia, except that, **without exception, horses affected with hepatic lipidosis must be on intravenous nutrition.** In addition, the veterinarian may chose to administer insulin, which slows the release of fat from the body cells. Heparin, a drug used to decrease the clotting ability of the blood, is also sometimes used to treat hepatic lipidosis as heparin also increases fat removal from the blood. Like hyperlipemia, the predisposing cause must be treated or eliminated.

PROGNOSIS

The prognosis for hyperlipemia and hepatic lipidosis is poor. Mortality rates have been estimated to be 60–100 percent with these diseases. [14, 15] The best chance for survival is when treatment is initiated at the first signs of hyperlipemia, before liver damage occurs.

PREVENTION

Prevention of these diseases is of critical importance because of the poor response to treatment.

- All horses should be on a diet that provides adequate nutrition, but does not induce obesity.
- Extreme stress should be avoided whenever possible, and horses that must be placed in a stressful situation should be closely monitored for depression or loss of appetite. Examples of stress-inducing situations include transportation, intense competition, late gestation, early lactation, and weaning.
- Any sickness or loss of appetite must be addressed immediately. The cause of the anorexia should be determined and treated. Every effort should be made to find a food that the horse will eat.

14 Naylor NG. Treatment and diagnosis of hyperlipemia and hyperlipidemia. Proc Am College of Vet Int Med; 1982: 47

15 Jeffcott LB, Field JR. Current concepts of hyperlipaemia in horses and ponies. *Vet Rec* 1985; 116: 461

- Blood work should be performed on sick or anorexia horses to monitor fat levels in the blood.
- Treatment should be initiated at the first the first signs of hyperlipemia.

Summary

Hyperlipemia and hepatic lipidosis are serious diseases that are often fatal. Miniature horses are at greater risk for these diseases than full-sized horses and should be monitored closely during times of illness or stress. Prevention is the most important step as treatment of these diseases is often not successful.

CHAPTER 6

The Endocrine System

THE ENDOCRINE SYSTEM is a complex interaction of organs and **hormones** that regulate the daily functions of the body. Various organs (thyroid gland, adrenal gland, pituitary gland, testicles, ovaries, etc.) manufacture and release hormones. These hormones are, in turn, taken up by other organs, which results in a change in activity or function of the receiving organ. For example, low levels of calcium in the blood stimulate the parathyroid gland (a small gland that sits next to the thyroid in the throat area) to secrete parathyroid hormone. This hormone causes a release of calcium from bone and an increase in absorption of calcium by the kidneys and intestines, thus returning blood calcium levels back to normal.

Endocrine disease is rare in horses of all breeds. Several diseases are worth mentioning with respect to Miniature horses, however, because they present special problems in management or diagnosis in this breed.

Cushing's Disease

CAUSE

Cushing's disease (pituitary adenoma) is caused by a tumor on the pituitary gland. It is generally a disease of old horses, but has been seen on rare occasion in younger animals. No predisposing factors for the formation of the tumor have been identified.

DIAGNOSIS

The pituitary gland produces and secretes several different hormones that have far reaching effects in the body. Therefore, the signs of Cushing's disease can be quite variable. The classic signs of the disease are a long hair coat that does not shed out, decreased energy levels, muscle wasting, and a pot-bellied appearance (figs. 6.1 A & B). Other signs that have been reported include increased drinking and urinating, dry scaly skin,

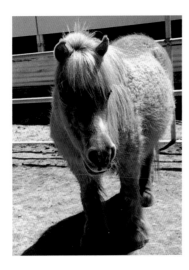

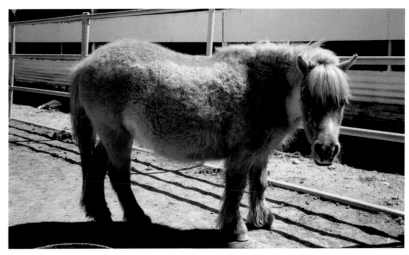

6.1 A & B A Miniature horse mare affected with Cushings disease. Note the long hair coat and potbelly. Wasting of the facial muscles gives her face a dished appearance.

increased susceptibility to infection, bulging of fat pads above the eyes, and intermittent colic. Horses with Cushing's disease are at increased risk for laminitis (see *Laminitis,* p. 11) and hepatic lipidosis (see *Hepatic Lipidosis,* p. 82).

The early signs of Cushing's disease are frequently missed in Miniature horses because of their tendency to have a long hair coat for much of the year. Also, many owners attribute the pot-bellied appearance of their older Miniature horses to obesity, when in fact the pot-bellied appearance to their abdomen is caused by abdominal muscle weakness secondary to the muscle wasting of Cushing's disease.

There are a number of tests used to diagnose Cushing's disease. The two most popular are measurement of cortisol levels in the blood and the dexamethasone suppression test.

Cortisol is a hormone secreted by the pituitary gland that helps regulate blood sugar levels. Normally, the pituitary gland secretes only enough cortisol to maintain an appropriate blood sugar level to meet the energy demands of the body. When the cortisol levels exceed what is needed for the animal's energy demands, the pituitary decreases its secretion of this hormone.

In Cushing's disease, the pituitary tumor secretes cortisol over and above what the body requires. These excess levels of cortisol can be measured in the blood to help diagnose the disease. The results of this test must be interpreted with caution as cortisol levels are increased in the morning hours and in response to exercise or stress. A normal cortisol level does not rule out the possibility of Cushing's disease and high cortisol levels can occur in normal, healthy horses.

A more accurate test for Cushing's disease is the dexamethasone suppression test. Dexamethasone is an injectable steroid that mimics cortisol in the bloodstream. A normal pituitary gland will decrease its secretion of cortisol when dexamethasone is administered. In this test, blood is taken for a baseline level of cortisol. The horse is then given an intravenous injection of dexamethasone. Several hours later, blood is redrawn for a post-injection cortisol level. In a normal horse, the level of cortisol in the blood will be less after the dexamethasone injection. In a horse with Cushing's disease, the cortisol level will remain high despite the administration of dexamethasone.

TREATMENT

The tumor that causes Cushing's disease cannot be removed surgically in horses. However, there are several medications that can be used to control the effects of the disease. Bromocriptine, pergolide, and cyproheptadine are medications that have been used with varying success to manage this disease. Thyroid dysfunction is sometimes seen with Cushing's disease and should be ruled out in any horse that is not responding to these treatments (see *Hypothyroidism,* below).

Careful management of horses with Cushing's disease is also important.

- Excess hair should be clipped in the warm weather.
- The horse should be housed in a clean environment and frequent grooming performed to prevent skin infections.
- Necessary precautions should be taken to prevent laminitis (see *Laminitis,* p. 11) and hepatic lipidosis (see *Hepatic Lipidosis,* p. 82).

PROGNOSIS

There is no cure for Cushing's disease. However, the medications currently available will control the effects of the disease in most cases. Treatment can make an old, tired, debilitated horse seem years younger and much happier.

Thyroid Abnormalities

The thyroid gland is responsible for regulating many of the functions of metabolism. The hormones secreted from the thyroid result in increased body temperature, oxygen consumption, protein synthesis, metabolic rate, heart rate, and nerve transmission.

Hypothyroidism
CAUSE

Hypothyroidism is a condition where inadequate amounts of thyroid hormone are produced or secreted. Reported causes of hypothyroidism in adult horses include iodine excess, iodine deficiency, thyroid tumors, and Cushing's disease. The main cause of hypothyroidism in foals is inadequate or excessive iodine intake by the mare during pregnancy and early lactation. Frequently, the underlying cause of hypothyroidism is not known.

Iodine deficiency in the diet is rare and usually seen only when the horse is being fed poor quality hay with no other dietary supplementation. Iodine excess can be a result of diet or related to absorption of other sources of iodine. Goiter (enlarged thyroid gland) has been seen in foals whose mares have been fed excessive amounts of iodine in kelp-supplemented rations. Other sources of iodine that have been suspected of causing iodine excess include leg paints, drugs (in particular, expectorants), and shampoos containing iodine.

DIAGNOSIS

Signs of hypothyroidism include weight gain, decreased energy levels, anemia, coarse hair coat, hair loss, irregular or absent **estrus** cycles in mares, and decreased libido in stallions. Because the thyroid gland plays a role in fat metabolism, hypothyroid horses are at greater risk for hepatic lipidosis than horses with normal thyroid function.

Hypothyroidism in foals is usually associated with goiter. Signs of hypothyroidism in foals are weakness, incoordination, defects in bone formation, forelimb contracture, long hair coat, and a poor suckle reflex. Hypothyroidism can be fatal in foals.

A preliminary diagnosis of hypothyroidism can be made by measuring the levels of thyroid hormone in the blood. However, thyroid hormone levels are affected by age, gender, drug administration, **systemic** illness, and normal daily variations. For example, thyroid hormone levels peak at about 4:00 PM and are at their lowest at 4:00 AM in most horses. If the blood levels are low, a second test is needed to confirm the diagnosis. The most commonly used test is the thyroid stimulating hormone (TSH) test. An initial baseline level of thyroid hormone is taken before administering a dose of TSH. In normal horses, there will be a marked increase in thyroid hormone levels within hours of administration of TSH. An inadequate response to TSH is an indication of thyroid dysfunction.

Caution: A horse should be off all medication for at least 30 days before performing either of these tests.

TREATMENT

Hypothyroidism can be treated by adding a thyroid supplement to the horse's diet. Most horses will need to stay on the treatment for the remainder of their lives. The horse should be monitored closely for signs of hyperthyroidism caused by over-supplementation. Iodine excesses or deficiencies should be corrected, but may not result in a reversal of the condition. Horses that do not respond as expected to thyroid supplementation should be evaluated for Cushing's disease as these conditions frequently go hand-in-hand.

Miniature horse owners should be aware of several points regarding hypothyroidism. Firstly, it is a rare disease in all horses. Weight gain in Miniatures is more frequently due to overfeeding as opposed to hypothyroidism. Secondly, because of their small size, all feed supplements should be used with care to avoid over-supplementation that could lead to the disease. Similarly, medications and shampoos with iodine should also be used with caution. Because of the difficulty estimating weight in Miniature horses, horses being treated with thyroid supplements should be monitored closely for signs of hyperthyroidism due to overdosing (see *Hyperthyroidism*, below). Finally, hypothyroid Miniature horses are at risk for the development of hepatic lipidosis and should be managed to prevent this serious complication (see *Hepatic Lipidosis*, p. 82).

PROGNOSIS

Most cases of hypothyroidism caused by iodine deficiency, or excess, can be successfully treated by addressing the underlying cause. In cases where the cause of the hypothyroidism is unknown, curing the disease is unlikely. Instead, the horse can be managed with thyroid supplementation. The prognosis is good for resolution of the clinical signs of the disease once an appropriate thyroid dose has been established.

Hyperthyroidism

CAUSE

Hyperthyroidism, a very rare disease in horses, is caused by excessive levels of thyroid hormones in the body. Excess exposure to iodine (feed, shampoos, leg paints, and drugs) and over-supplementation with thyroid hormone are the most common causes of this disease.

DIAGNOSIS

The signs of hyperthyroidism are due to the elevated metabolism that occurs with increase thyroid hormone levels and include high heart rate, excitability, tremors, sweating, and weight loss despite a good appetite. High blood levels of thyroid hormone are diagnostic of the disease. High thyroid hormone levels are also seen in normal foals and pregnant mares. Therefore, hyperthyroidism should only be suspected in these horses if they are showing signs of the disease.

Treatment of hyperthyroidism is directed at removing the excess source of iodine or decreasing the dose of thyroid supplement. Return to normal may not be immediate, but will occur as the excess iodine is processed. Iodine containing feed supplements, shampoos, leg paints, and medications should be used with caution in Miniature horses. Horses that are on thyroid supplements should be monitored closely for signs of hyperthyroidism. Periodic measurement of blood thyroid levels is recommended in horses being treated for hypothyroidism with thyroid hormone supplements.

PROGNOSIS

If the underlying cause of the hyperthyroidism can be determined and eliminated, there is a good prognosis that the disease can be cured.

Summary

Endocrine disorders are relatively rare in Miniature horses, but should be considered any time there is a change in a horse's body condition, energy level, or temperament. Treatment of these abnormalities is usually successful and can make a huge difference in an animal's quality of life, as well as preventing more serious, secondary diseases such as laminitis and hepatic lipidosis.

CHAPTER 7

Reproduction

WITH THE EVER-INCREASING popularity and value of Miniature horses, the importance of well-managed breeding programs cannot be overemphasized. Proper care and management of stallions, broodmares, and neonatal foals allows for increased productivity and better health for the animals. The goal of every breeding program should be to produce individuals that not only meet the breed standard but also add to the quality of the breed as a whole.

There are several differences between Miniature horses and full-sized horses in the area of reproduction. The small size of the Miniature horse requires special considerations regarding equipment for semen collection, evaluation of semen, and the use of rectal and ultrasound examinations for evaluation of the mare's reproductive tract. Miniature horse mares appear to be more prone to abortions and difficult deliveries than full-sized mares. Therefore, breeders should be aware of the signs of a problem and be prepared to deal with the emergency appropriately.

The Stallion

In general, there are few differences between Miniature horse stallions and full sized stallions. Problems with libido and fertility appear to be rare in the Miniature horses. However, there are certain points with respect to evaluation and management of Miniature horse stallions that are worth discussion.

Cryptorchidism

Normal Testicular Descent
In the early stages of fetal development, the testes are located within the abdomen. It is not until the fetus is between 270 and 300 days old that the

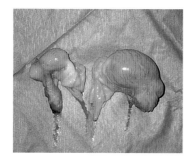

7.1 (above) Testicles removed from a cryptorchid stallion. The testicle on the left was retained in the abdomen, while the testicle on the right was in a normal scrotal position. Notice the smaller size of the retained testicle.

7.2 (right) An artificial vagina (AV).

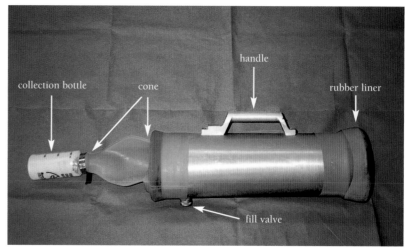

testicle begins to pass out of the abdomen, through an opening in the abdominal wall called the **inguinal canal** (a slit in the abdominal wall located in the groin area at the top of the thigh), into the scrotum.

Cryptorchid

A *cryptorchid* is a male animal whose testicle has not descended from the abdomen into its normal position in the scrotum. The testicle may be located in the abdomen, inguinal canal, or external to the inguinal canal. Cryptorchid testicles are small and poorly developed and their sperm production is decreased or absent (fig. 7.1). One or both testicles can be affected. If one normal testicle is present, the horse will be fertile due to the presence of the scrotal testicle, but should not be bred as cryporchidism is considered to be a genetic defect.

Many colts have temporary retention of one or both testicles external and adjacent to the inguinal canal. Most of these testicles will descend into the scrotum when they have matured in size; therefore, these horses are not true cryptorchids.

DIAGNOSIS

The diagnosis of cryptorchidism is easily reached by **palpation** of the scrotal sac. The challenge lies in determining the location of the testicle that is not present in the scrotum. Testicles in the abdomen or inguinal canal cannot be palpated. Those that are external to the canal can sometimes be located with careful palpation of the inguinal area. Sedation will relax the colt, allowing a more thorough palpation. An ultrasound exam will sometimes help to locate the testicle. Even with the use of sedation, careful palpation, and

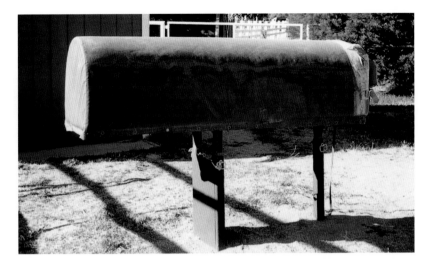

7.3 A full-sized horse dummy mount. The stallion's penis is directed into the artificial vagina (AV) after he mounts the dummy. A scaled-down version of the dummy mount can be made to use with Miniature horse stallions.

ultrasonography, it may be difficult to locate the testicle. This is especially true in Miniature horses where the retained testicle is very small and a layer of fat is often present in the inguinal area.

If a colt is of quality to be a breeding stallion, but one or both testicles have not descended into the scrotum, the best approach may be to wait and see. Male Miniature horses with undescended testicles can be shown in AMHA-recognized shows up to three years of age. The horse should not be bred during this waiting period in case he is a true cryptorchid. If the testicle has not reached the scrotum by three years of age, the horse should be considered a cryptorchid and should be castrated.

Cryptorchid castration is more complicated, therefore more expensive, than castration of a colt with both testicles in the scrotum. Frequently, the abdomen must be entered to retrieve the testicle. Therefore, many veterinarians prefer to perform the surgery in a surgery suite as opposed to field castration.

Semen Collection

Collection of semen is necessary for reproductive evaluations and artificial insemination. Usually, an artificial vagina (AV) (fig. 7.2) is used for collection, although some stallion handlers have collected their stallions using a condom or trained them to ejaculate into a collection bottle or bag with manual stimulation.

When collecting a stallion with an artificial vagina, a mare in estrus (in heat) or a dummy mount is used for the stallion to mount. A dummy is a canvas, vinyl, or leather-covered padded stand that looks similar to a gymnastic vaulting horse (fig. 7.3). Some training is necessary in order to get a stallion to mount a dummy. After the stallion mounts the mare or dummy, the penis is directed into the AV.

Care should be used when purchasing a dummy or AV for use in collection of Miniature horse stallions. The dummy must be made especially for Miniature horses. Dummies made for ponies may be short enough, but are usually too wide for a Miniature horse to straddle comfortably. The height of the dummy should be at about the height of the tail head of the stallion when standing, and a width of 12–14 inches is comfortable for most Miniature horses.[16]

It is very important to use an AV that is short enough so that the stallion ejaculates into the cone, not the lining of the AV. The lining of an AV is filled with very warm water to stimulate the stallion to ejaculate (111 to 122 degrees Fahrenheit; 44 to 50 degrees Centigrade). This temperature will kill sperm if the semen comes into contact with the inside of the AV before passing through the cone and into the collection bottle.

Commercially manufactured AVs for ponies and Miniature horses are shorter than those made for full-sized horses to accommodate the shorter penis. However, most of these are as wide as those made for full-sized stallions. That makes it difficult to generate enough warm water pressure in the AV for some Miniature horse stallions to be sufficiently stimulated to ejaculate.

There are several solutions to these problems. An AV can be constructed using PVC piping. This allows production of an AV with the length and width appropriate for a Miniature horse stallion (fig. 7.4).[17] If the wider, commercial AV is used and the stallion does not ejaculate, additional stimulation by the application of warm towels to the base of the penis while the stallion is thrusting will sometimes induce ejaculation.

Because of the lack of appropriate equipment for collection of semen from Miniature horse stallions, some handlers prefer to collect stallions through the use of manual stimulation with the stallion standing or mounted on a mare.[18] Most stallions will readily accept this technique with proper training. The quantity and quality of collected semen is unaffected by the use of this method.[19]

---

16 Instructions on how to build a dummy mount can be obtained from Dr. Sue McDonnell of the Equine Behavior Lab at the University of Pennsylvania School of Veterinary Medicine. See Appendix D.

17 Instructions on building a Miniature horse AV can be obtained from FA Ranch and Racing. See Appendix D.

18 Forney, BD, McDonnell SM. How to Collect Semen from Stallions While They Are Standing on the Ground. 45th Annu Conv Am Assoc Equine Practnr 1999; 142

19 McDonnell SM, Love CC. Manual stimulation collection of semen from stallions: Training time, sexual behavior and semen. *Theriogenology,*; 33: 1201

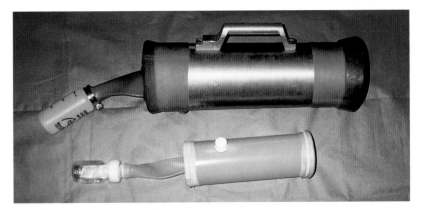

7.4 A homemade Miniature horse artificial vagina (AV) shown next to a full-sized horse one for size comparison. (Miniature horse AV: courtesy of FA Ranch and Racing, Reno, NV).

The stallion can also be fitted with a nonspermicidal human condom. Breeders that have used this method report that the stallion accepts the condom well and have not had a problem with it becoming dislodged in the mare.[20] Obviously, a mare in heat is necessary for collection and it is important that the penis is very clean before application and the semen is filtered before evaluation or use. Filtration is especially important if an automated counter is used to obtain a sperm count, as particulate matter will interfere with the results.

Reproductive Evaluation

Reproductive evaluation of a stallion is generally performed before the purchase or sale of the individual. Other reasons for a reproductive evaluation include estimation of the number of mares that can be covered in a season; estimating the number of breedings per day a stallion can manage without reduced fertility; anytime the stallion exhibits abnormal sexual behavior; or anytime there is a suspicion that a stallion's fertility may changed, such as after an illness.

The stallion's libido and ability to mount and cover a mare are assessed during the reproductive evaluation. Testicular size is measured as it reflects the potential sperm-producing ability of the stallion (larger testicles produce more sperm). In addition, semen is collected and evaluated for the number, appearance, and motility of sperm in the ejaculate. The semen should be cultured for infectious agents.

There is no significant difference between Miniature horse stallions and full-sized stallions with respect to the appearance and motility of sperm. However, Miniature horse stallions' testicles are smaller and therefore produce less volume of semen and fewer sperm per ejaculation than full-sized stallions. Therefore, normal parameters that have been calculated in full-sized stallions cannot be used to evaluate Miniature horse stallions.

In order to predict fertility in Miniature horse stallions, Drs. Metcalf, Ley, and Love collected semen from twenty-three Miniature horse stallions that were known to be fertile.[21] The average left and right testicular volumes were 30.61 cubic centimeters and 31.91 cubic centimeters, respectively. The average seminal volume in an ejaculate was 17.0 milliliters with an average sperm concentration of 177.2 million sperm/milliliter and an average total number of sperm per ejaculate of 2 billion. These numbers provide a guideline by which to compare Miniature horse stallions when evaluating their potential fertility.

Artificial Insemination

The most common method of breeding Miniature horses is still live or natural cover. However, as the AMHA now allows registration of foals conceived by artificial insemination, this method of reproduction will likely gain in popularity.

Advantages of Artificial Insemination
There are several advantages to artificial insemination over natural cover. Artificial insemination is safer for both the mare and the stallion, especially if a dummy mount or manual stimulation is used to collect the stallion. Not only is the risk of injury to the animals decreased, but the risk of transmission of infection between horses is greatly reduced. Also, because a single ejaculate can be divided into multiple insemination doses, a stallion can breed more mares per season. Finally, as semen can be shipped across the country, artificial insemination provides a means for greater genetic variation in the breed, as the choice of stallions is not limited to those in close proximity to a mare.

Disadvantages of Artificial Insemination
The disadvantages of artificial insemination are the expense of the necessary equipment, and the greater degree of knowledge and skill needed for a successful breeding program. After collection, the semen must be appropriately

---

21 Metcalf ES, Ley WB, Love CC. Semen parameters of the American miniature horse stallion. 43rd Annu Conv Am Assoc Equine Practnr 1997; 202

handled and processed in order for the sperm to survive. Also, the mare must be closely monitored to ensure insemination within twenty-four to seventy-two hours before ovulation. Any breeding establishment wishing to incorporate artificial insemination should work closely with a veterinarian or trained technician in order to ensure that current best practices are being followed.

AMHA Regulations

The American Miniature Horse Association has placed several limitations on the use of artificial insemination. A foal conceived using artificial insemination can only be registered with the AMHA and AMHR if the following criteria have been met: [22]

- Artificial insemination was performed using cooled, NOT FROZEN semen.
- The mare was on the same premises as the stallion and was immediately bred (within twenty-four hours) with the collected semen.
- If the mare was not on the premises and the semen was shipped to her, the stallion must have had a transported semen permit for the year in which the foal was conceived. Blood/DNA genetic testing of the stallion must be on record with the AMHA before a permit is issued.
- Insemination of any mare bred with shipped semen was performed within seventy-two hours of collection of the semen.
- The stallion did not breed more than a total of twenty mares by artificial insemination during the season the foal was conceived.
- A collection-insemination report was filed by the mare owner.
- The foal's parentage has been verified using blood/DNA testing of the mare and foal.

Equine Viral Arteritis and the Breeding Stallion

Equine viral arteritis (EVA) is a contagious disease of horses caused by a virus. Some infected horses develop no clinical signs of disease whereas in other horses EVA can cause fever; depression; loss of appetite; swelling of the face, legs, mammary glands and genitals; nasal discharge; pneumonia; abortion of pregnant mares; and death of young foals. An EVA outbreak on a breeding farm can be devastating to the existing foals as well as the next, unborn foal crop.

---

22 These regulations were taken from the 2002 AMHA Rule Book. Breeders should consult their breed association or registry regarding current regulations on the use of artificial insemination. While the AMHR rulebook does not discuss the use of artificial insemination, horses registered with the AMHA are eligible for registration with the AMHR.

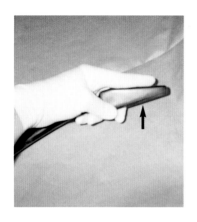

7.5 An ultrasound probe. The probe is held in the veterinarian's hand as shown and inserted into the rectum. Ultrasound waves are transmitted from and received by the surface of the probe (arrow), which is placed on the floor of the rectum. The returned waves are converted into an image by the ultrasound machine.

Stallions can be carriers of this disease without showing any clinical signs. If a carrier stallion passes the virus to an unvaccinated mare through natural cover or artificial insemination, she can develop the disease and pass it on to the mares and foals in which she comes into contact. For this reason, the American Association of Equine Practitioners (AAEP) recommends that all breeding stallions be tested for EVA.

While EVA outbreaks in Miniature horses have not been reported, in the study by Metcalf, Ley, and Love see footnote [21], 8.7 percent of the stallions tested positive for the virus. Therefore, testing of Miniature horses that will be used as breeding stallions is advised.

A vaccine is available to protect horses against EVA. There are several guidelines that should be followed when using the vaccine. Horses should be tested for EVA before administration of the vaccine. Pregnant or nursing mares should not be vaccinated. Vaccinated animals should be isolated for twenty-one days as shedding of the virus is possible post-vaccination. Because of the complexities in using this vaccine, breeders should contact their veterinarian to discuss if vaccination is appropriate for their animals.

The Mare

Rectal Examination and Ultrasonography

In full-sized mares, rectal and ultrasound examinations play a crucial role in the majority of breeding programs. These techniques are useful for evaluating the reproductive health of the mare, following the estrus cycle, pregnancy detection, and monitoring fetal health.

During a rectal examination, the veterinarian removes any feces present in the rectum. A hand is then inserted and the reproductive tract is palpated (felt) through the wall of the rectum. The degree of relaxation of the cervix, the size and tone of the uterus, and the presence of follicles on the ovaries can be determined.

Rectal examinations are often combined with ultrasonographic examination of the reproductive organs. It is important that manure be completely cleared from the rectum before the ultrasound exam as fecal material will interfere with visualization of the reproductive structures.

The ultrasound machine creates waves that are transmitted from a probe, which is held in the veterinarian's hand and placed on the floor of the rectum (fig. 7.5). The waves bounce off the soft-tissue structures and return to the probe. The machine then converts the returned waves to a picture that

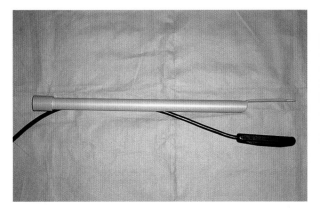

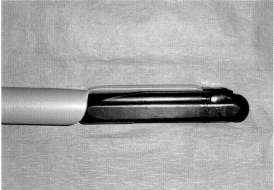

is projected onto a monitor. This provides a visual, real-time image of the uterus, ovaries, and pregnancy. This is called transrectal ultrasonography because the image is taken through the wall of the rectum.

Transrectal ultrasonography of the reproductive tract allows identification of uterine abnormalities, such as fluid in the uterus (an indication of infection) and uterine cysts (which can possibly affect fertility), visualization of ovarian activity including pending ovulation, and early detection of pregnancy. Ultrasound can also be used through the wall of the abdomen (transabdominal) to visualize pregnancies. This is most accurate when the pregnancy is greater than sixty days of gestation.

Rectal examinations and transrectal ultrasonography have not been used as commonly in Miniature mares as in full-sized mares. This is because of the Miniature horse's small size and the possibility of an accidental rectal tear. Rectal tearing is a risk even in full-sized mares, but is even more of a concern in Miniature horse mares. However, as more and more Miniature horse breeders have adopted intensive management protocols for their breeding programs, the need for these diagnostics has become apparent and the veterinary profession has developed ways to safely provide this service.

Veterinarians with small or average-sized hands and forearms can in most cases safely perform rectal examinations and transrectal ultrasounds in Miniature horses. The mare must be properly restrained either in stocks or with sedation. Any mare that is struggling or straining excessively should be sedated. Infusion of the rectum with lidocaine (a numbing agent similar to novacaine) will help relax the rectum of a straining mare.

If the veterinarian's hands or forearms are large or the mare is very small or uncooperative, it is better not to risk rectal injury by introduction of a hand into the rectum. However, with the use of a probe handle extension (figs. 7.6 A & B), it is possible to perform an ultrasound exam. The mare is

7.6 A (left) A probe handle extension and ultrasound probe before the probe is taped into position.

7.6 B (above)
The probe has been inserted into the probe handle extension. It is then taped into place, lubricated, and inserted into the mare's rectum.

given an enema to clear feces from the rectum. The ultrasound probe is placed into a probe handle extension[23], which is then inserted into the rectum and used to visualize the reproductive tract. The mare should be appropriately restrained to prevent injury to the rectal wall by the probe. There is less control over the positioning of the probe with the handle extension; therefore, visualization of the entire reproductive tract can be difficult.

The veterinarian should make the decision as to which approach is used to evaluate a mare. Factors that affect that choice include the size and temperament of the mare, the size of the veterinarian's arms and hands, the ability to restrain the mare, and the farm's approach to breeding management.

The Estrous Cycle

Estrus is the period when a mare is sexually receptive. The term "in heat" is frequently used by horsemen to describe this period. The estrous cycle is the period from estrus to estrus. Mares are seasonally polyestrous, meaning that they have multiple estrous cycles during the spring, summer, and fall. Because of the short periods of daylight in the winter, mares enter an anestrous period where they do not cycle.

The estrous cycle lasts an average of twenty-one days in most mares with the mare being in heat for only five to seven of those days. Ovulation, the release of an egg from the ovary, usually occurs one to two days before the end of estrus. The greatest possibility of pregnancy is achieved if the mare is bred twenty-four to seventy-eight hours before ovulation. If the egg is not fertilized, the mare will return to estrus about fourteen to eighteen days after ovulation.

Detection of Estrus
Recognizing when a mare is in estrus is crucial to a successful breeding. One approach to estrus detection is a process called teasing. Teasing a mare involves exposing the mare to a stallion and watching her behavior. Behavioral signs of estrus include interest in the stallion, tail raising, squatting, urinating, and "winking" of the vulva (retraction of the vulvar lips to expose the clitoris). When a mare is not in estrus she will ignore the stallion or even show aggressive behavior toward him.

Detection of estrus becomes much more difficult if a stallion is not available. This may be the case if artificial insemination is being performed with shipped semen. Some mares will demonstrate changes in their normal behavior during estrus and may even tease to a gelding or another mare. If

---

23 Classic Medical Supply, Inc. See Appendix D.

a stallion is not available and the mare does not show behavioral signs of estrus, rectal or ultrasound examinations can be used to follow a mare through her cycle. One exam is rarely adequate to determine the stage of a mare's cycle. Instead, multiple examinations are needed to determine when a mare is coming into estrus.

When ultrasound is not available and the mare's size precludes the use of rectal examinations, the cervix can be monitored to determine estrus. The cervix becomes soft, wet, and open when the mare is in estrus. This can be determined through digital palpation (a mare's vagina is much tougher and has greater stretch than her rectum) or by using a small vaginal speculum (a section of PVC pipe that is eight-to-ten-inches long and one or two inches in diameter can be used. The end must be beveled and smoothed to prevent injury to the vagina.). The mare and examiner must be thoroughly cleaned and all instruments sterilized to prevent the introduction of infection into the mare's reproductive tract.

Anestrus

Anestrus is a term used to describe sexual inactivity in a mare. A mare in anestrus will show no signs of a normal estrus cycle. In true anestrus, the ovaries are not functional and are not producing the hormones responsible for cycling. Seasonal anestrus occurs in mares during the winter months and is a normal condition. Anestrus during the spring and summer months is an abnormal condition and may be a result of ovarian disease or malfunction, old age, Cushing's disease, or hypothyroidism (see *Endocrine System,* p. 85).

Behavioral anestrus, also called "silent heat," is condition where the mare has normal ovarian function and cyclic hormonal changes, but is not receptive to the stallion. This is more common in maiden mares (mares that have never had a foal), nervous or shy mares, and mares with a foal at their side.

Some veterinarians believe that anestrus is more common in Miniature horses than in full-sized mares. If a mare is not cycling as expected, she should be examined by a veterinarian. Repeat ultrasonography of the reproductive tract or repeat measurement of blood hormone levels may be necessary to distinguish true anestrus from behavioral anestrus.

Examination of the cervix may also be helpful. If the cervix is wet and relaxed but the mare is not receptive to the stallion, she is probably demonstrating behavioral anestrus. On the other hand, a consistently closed cervix in conjunction with anestrus behavior is a good indication that the mare is not cycling.

If the mare is not showing estrus activity, careful ultrasound examination of the ovaries should be performed if possible (see *Rectal Examination and Ultrasonography,* p. 98). Tests to rule out Cushing's disease and hypothyroidism may also need to be performed (see *Endocrine System,* Chapter Six). It is also important to be sure that the mare is not pregnant as this is a common reason for anestrus behavior.

If the mare has normal ovarian activity, but is not interested in the stallion management changes may help the mare be more receptive. The mare should be given plenty of time to adjust to her surroundings and the stallion. A standard routine for teasing should be used to allow the mare to become familiar with the process. Some mares tease better in a group, while others prefer to be exposed to the stallion alone. Timid mares will often respond better to less aggressive stallions or may not appear receptive when the stallion is close, but will show signs of estrus when allowed to move away from the stallion. Some mares with foals will only show signs of heat if the foal is out of view whereas others only show signs when the foal is at her side. If a handler is willing to try different approaches to teasing and is patient and observant, estrus may be detected in these mares.

In summary, the first step in managing an anestrus mare is to determine if she is in true anestrus or behavioral anestrus. If a mare is not cycling due to inactivity or malfunctioning of her ovaries, every attempt should be made to find the reason, as treatment of the primary cause will often allow the mare to return to estrus. If the mare is displaying behavioral anestrus, the first step is to try changing how the mare is teased or using a different stallion. If the mare continues to be nonreceptive, following ovarian activity or cervical changes may be the only alternative. Once the mare has been determined to be in estrus, natural cover may be attempted with proper restraint of the mare. If the mare resists all attempts at natural cover, she can be bred with artificial insemination.

Gestation (Pregnancy)

Gestation is the period from fertilization of the egg until the foal is born. The gestation period in horses is 320–360 days, although some Miniature horse breeders have reported gestation lengths as short as 310 days.

Detection of Pregnancy
Teasing
The most basic approach to pregnancy detection is to continue to tease the mare and assume she is pregnant if she no longer shows behavioral signs of estrus. The problem with this is that non-pregnant mares may have behavioral anestrus and some pregnant mares will continue to show signs of heat when teased by a stallion. For these reasons, while

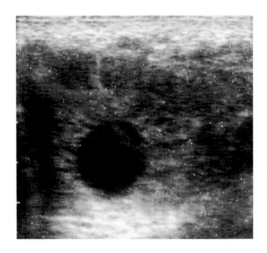

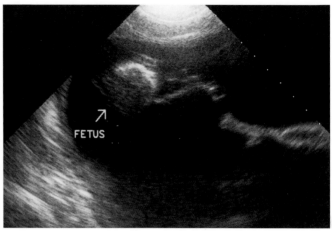

teasing is the simplest method of pregnancy detection, it is not the most reliable.

Teasing can be combined with examination of the cervix. The cervix is tightly closed in a pregnant mare and a closed cervix provides additional proof of pregnancy in a mare that does not show signs of estrus after breeding. If the cervix is relaxed, it is unlikely that the mare is pregnant, even if she shows no sexual interest in the stallion. It is important that examination of the cervix, whether performed with a hand or speculum, be done gently as trauma to the cervix can cause the mare to abort. Also, strict cleanliness on the part of the examiner is vital to prevent the introduction of infectious agents that could lead to abortion.

Rectal Examination
If the veterinarian feels that it can be performed safely, rectal examination can be used for diagnosing pregnancy. In full-sized horses, pregnancy can be reliably detected by rectal palpation alone after thirty days of gestation. Because of the small size of the pregnancy, rectal palpation at thirty days is not as reliable in Miniature horses and repeat palpations may need to be performed at forty-five or sixty days for a more accurate determination.

Ultrasound Examination
The accuracy of pregnancy detection can be greatly increased with the use of transrectal ultrasound. This can be performed with the hand in the rectum holding the probe or by the use of a probe handle extension (see *Rectal Examination and Ultrasonography*, p. 98). An experienced veterinarian can reliably diagnose a pregnancy with transrectal ultrasonography in a Miniature horse by eighteen days of gestation (fig. 7.7).

7.7 (left) An ultrasound image of an eighteen-day pregnancy in a Miniature horse mare.

7.8 (right) A transabdominal ultrasound image of a sixty-day Miniature horse pregnancy.

Transabdominal ultrasound can also be used to diagnose a pregnancy. Because the ultrasound must penetrate through more tissue, the pregnancy must be older and therefore larger than what can be detected with transrectal examination. Veterinarians experienced in the use of transabdominal ultrasound can detect pregnancy as early as thirty days in Miniature horses, but examination at forty-five to sixty days is more reliable (fig. 7.8)

Hormone Levels

Blood hormone levels have been investigated as a means for early pregnancy diagnosis in Miniature horses. In full-sized mares, estrone sulfate, a type of estrogen, is elevated after seventy days of gestation and is a reliable indicator of pregnancy. Unfortunately, estrone sulfate levels are not a reliable indicator of pregnancy in Miniature horses.

Investigators have developed a protocol for measuring hormones in Miniature horses that is very reliable for pregnancy detection.[24] In this method, an increase in equine chorionic gonadotropin (a hormone synthesized and secreted by the placenta) to over 300 nanograms/milliliter in combination with an increase in estrone sulfate between forty-five and sixty days after breeding is diagnostic of pregnancy. Measurement of either of these hormones alone is not a reliable means to detect pregnancy.

Abortion

CAUSES

Miniature horse mares appear to be at greater risk for abortion than full-sized mares. Many of these abortions are late term (after six months of gestation) and are frequently associated with a malformed fetus.

In addition to fetal malformation, there are many other possible causes of abortion including twinning, twisting of the umbilical cord, separation of the placenta from the uterine wall, and bacterial, fungal, or viral infections of the placenta and/or fetus. The placenta and fetus should be examined by a veterinarian to try to determine the cause of the abortion so that measures can be taken to prevent repeat abortion in the affected mare or spread of infection to other mares in the herd. If the abortion was caused by bacterial or fungal infection, the mare may need to be treated before attempting another breeding.

The association between genetics and abortion of a malformed fetus has not been proven. However, as these deformities may be related to dwarfism,

---

24 Foristall KM, Roser JF, Liu IKM, Lasley B, Munro CJ, Carneiro GF. Development of a tandem hormone assay for the detection of pregnancy in the miniature mare. 44th Annu Conv Am Assoc Equine Practnr 1998; 52

it may be wise to not repeat a breeding that has resulted in an abortion due to malformation (see p. 00 [Chapter 9]).

A common cause of abortion in horses of all breeds is equine herpesvirus type 1 (EHV 1) infection. This virus is highly contagious and causes respiratory infection, neurologic disease, and abortions in horses. Prevention of this disease involves proper management practices and vaccination.

PREVENTION

New arrivals to a breeding farm should be isolated from the pregnant mare herd. Many farms require that all incoming animals be vaccinated against EHV 1. Overcrowding and stress should be avoided in pregnant mares. If an animal becomes infected, its environment should be considered contaminated for three weeks. The movement of pregnant mares to new environments, such as in showing, should be avoided.

A vaccine is available to help prevent EHV 1 abortions.[25] It is administered at five, seven, and nine months of gestation, and when combined with proper management practices, will help decrease the incidence of abortion due to this disease. Many Miniature horse breeders are under the mistaken impression that this vaccine is not safe for Miniature horses. They feel that the vaccine can cause abortion. At this time there is no scientific evidence that this is true. More likely, because Miniature horse mares are at higher risk for abortion, the abortion coincidentally occurred near the same time as the vaccination and the vaccination was wrongly accused of causing the abortion. Consultation with a veterinarian before administration of any vaccine is recommended if a mare has had any type of vaccination reactions in the past.

Prenatal Care

It is important that the mare receives good nutrition and health care during the pregnancy. As the needs of the mare vary with the geographical area and management practices of the farm, the best approach is for the breeder to consult with his veterinarian to plan gestational care. For example, pasture and hay in many states is typically very low in selenium, so that selenium supplementation of mares in these areas is critical. As Miniature horses in general are easy keepers, mares should be monitored closely for excessive weight gain during pregnancy.

Pregnant mares should be housed separately from the general horse population to minimize their exposure to infectious disease. This is especially

---

25 Prodigy, Intervet Inc; Pneumabort-K + 1b, Fort Dodge Animal Health. See Appendix D.

important on farms where new horses are frequently introduced or horses come and go as part of a showing schedule.

Vaccination against EHV 1 at five, seven, and nine months of pregnancy is recommended (see *Abortion,* p. 104). A complete set of routine vaccinations should be given four to six weeks before the mare's predicted foaling date. This not only provides increased protection to the mare during this stressful period, but mares vaccinated late in pregnancy produce higher quality **colostrum** (the first milk that provides protective antibodies to the foal) rich in antibodies. The choice of vaccines is affected by the area of the country, and the farm's management practices. A veterinarian should be consulted as to which vaccines are appropriate for each particular mare. The veterinarian should be made aware of any reactions, such as fever, depression, swelling at the site of injection, or swelling of her legs, that a mare has had to previous vaccination.

The mare naturally produces antibodies against infectious agents in her environment. It takes several weeks for a mare to produce an antibody against a new agent in her environment. Therefore, it is recommended that the environment of the mare not be changed during the last four weeks of pregnancy. In this way, the foal is provided with colostrum containing antibodies against those infectious agents to which it will be exposed. If a mare will be foaling at a different location from where she is housed during her pregnancy, she should be moved to that location four to six weeks before her expected delivery date.

Mares should not be grazed on fescue grass pasture or fed fescue grass hay during the last month of pregnancy. Fescue is frequently infected with an endophyte (a fungal parasite of the grass). Ingestion of endophyte-infected fescue can cause prolonged gestation, placental abnormalities, abortion, weak foals, or lack of milk production. If a mare has accidentally ingested fescue during her last month of pregnancy, a veterinarian should be consulted as to proper management of this high-risk pregnancy.

Because of the risk of late-term abortion in Miniature horse mares, frequent observation of mares in their last trimester of pregnancy is recommended. Many late-term abortions are due to a malformed fetus. The deformity may make it difficult for the fetus to pass through the birth canal. Assisted delivery of these fetuses may be necessary to prevent an injury to the mare that could affect her fertility.

Miniature horse mares in late gestation and early lactation are at increased risk for the development of hyperlipemia and hepatic lipidosis (see *Hyperlipemia,* p. 79 and *Hepatic Lipidosis,* p. 82). Veterinary examination is recommended if a mare becomes depressed or loses her appetite, both early signs of these diseases.

Parturition (Birthing)

Preparation

Signs of impending **parturition** include filling of the udder and teats, waxing of the teats (a wax-like droplet forms on the teat opening), and relaxation of the vulva and muscles in the tail area. The constituents of the secretions in the mammary gland change as parturition approaches, and there are multiple commercially available test kits that measure the electrolyte concentration in the mare's milk to predict the mare's readiness to foal.[26]

Once it is determined that the mare is nearing parturition, she should be monitored around the clock. Electronic monitoring systems that are attached to the mare and set off an alarm when the mare goes into labor are available.[27] Complete reliance on these systems is not recommended as any technical or mechanical failure of the system could result in a mare going into labor unattended. In addition, monitoring systems that are attached to the vulvar lips and triggered by the foal beginning to pass out the vagina, will not be activated if the foal is malpositioned in the uterus. Such a foal will not pass far enough out of the uterus to trip the alarm.

In preparation for foaling, the mare's udder should be cleaned with warm water and dried well. The area between the mammary glands tends to collect dirt and should receive special attention. This procedure also allows first-time mothers to become accustomed to having their teats touched. A tail wrap should be applied and the vulva and surrounding area cleaned. These hygiene practices are important to decrease the foal's exposure to infectious agents as it searches for the nipple during its first attempts to nurse.

Ideally, foaling should take place in a quiet, roomy stall with straw bedding, but foaling on a grass pasture is also acceptable as long as the mare is supervised and other horses are not present to worry her. Foaling on shavings should be avoided, as there appears to be an association between the development of pneumonia in the foal and bedding on shavings.

Stages of Labor

There are three stages of parturition in the horse. In Stage I, uterine contractions help to position the foal so that its back is pointed up and the front legs and head are extended, which is the normal birthing position. Signs of Stage I labor include restlessness, pacing, tail switching, the mare looking at her side, sweating, frequent recumbency, and frequent passing of small

---

[26] Predict–A–Foal, Animal Health Care Products. See Appendix D.

[27] foalert, foalert, Inc. See Appendix D.

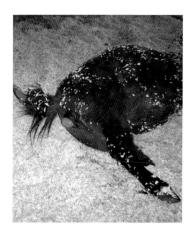

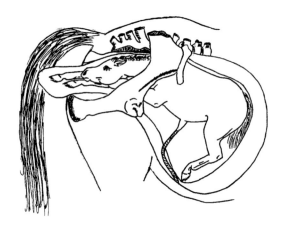

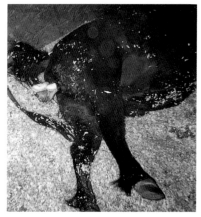

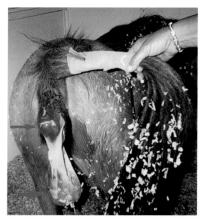

7.9 (above) The amniotic sac should become visible soon after contractions begin. It is easily identified as a slippery, gray-white membrane (Photo courtesy of Kitty and Bill Pearce).

7.10 A (above right) The normal presentation of a foal for delivery.

7.10 B (near right) The normal position of the feet at first presentation. One foot is slightly behind the other, with both feet pointing downward (Photo courtesy of Kitty and Bill Pearce).

7.11 (far right) This delivery is progressing normally. The front legs are well out, with the feet pointing downward (see large arrow). The nose (small arrow) is positioned at the level of the foal's carpi. Notice that the amniotic sac is still intact (Photo courtesy of Vickie Swaroski).

7.12 The mare will usually rest for several minutes with the foal's legs still in the birth canal. Notice that the mare is already bonding with the foal (Photo courtesy of Vickie Swaroski).

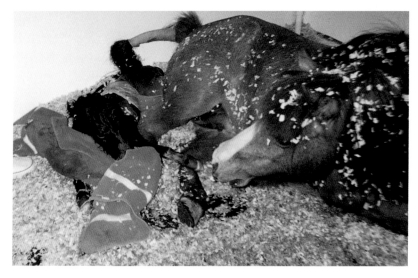

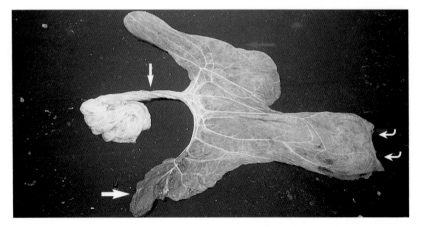

7.13 A completely passed placenta should have an umbilical cord (see small white arrow), an intact gravid horn where the foal was carried (red arrow), an intact nongravid horn (large white arrow), and an opening where the foal ruptured the placenta during delivery (curved arrows).

amounts of feces and urine. Stage I labor can persist for hours or even days and can easily be interrupted if the mare becomes anxious or excited.

Stage II labor begins with the rupture of the placenta and passing of the allantoic fluid ("breaking water"). The mare may change positions several times and multiple contractions occur before the foal in its amniotic (fetal) sac becomes visible. The amniotic sac is easily recognized as a gray-white slippery membrane (fig. 7.9).

The normal presentation of the foal is with one foot slightly behind the other and the nose resting on top of, or to the side of the legs at about the level of the foal's carpi. The bottom of the feet should be pointing downward (figs. 7.10 A & B, and 7.11). Most mares foal lying on their side, but some will give birth while standing. If the mare attempts to deliver standing, an assistant should be ready to catch the foal before it hits the ground.

Stage II labor ends when the foal's hips clear the mare's pelvis. If the amniotic sac covering the foal's nose does not break as the foal passes through the birth canal, it should be opened as soon as the nose becomes visible.

Stage II labor should be relatively rapid with the average time from breaking water and birth of the foal lasting about twenty minutes. Stage II labor that continues for more than thirty minutes may be an indication that there is a problem with the delivery.

Usually, the mare lies quietly for several minutes after the foal is born, often with the foal's rear legs still in the birth canal (fig. 7.12). Eventually she will stand and begin examining and licking the foal. If the mare and foal appear to be stable, it is important that they be disturbed as little as possible during this time in order for the mare and foal to bond to each other. A nervous mare or first-time mother may reject the foal if there is too much activity or too many people present during this critical period.

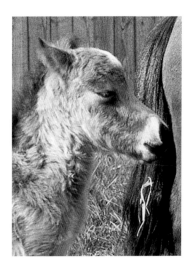

7.14 A two-day-old Miniature horse foal. Notice the prominent dome on his forehead that is found in most neonatal Miniature horses. This dome can lead to a difficult delivery if the foal is relatively large compared to the mare.

Stage III labor is the passing of the placental membranes. The mare will continue to have contractions during this stage and may paw, pace, and roll. The placenta should pass within three hours of the birth of the foal and should be examined to be sure that none of it has been retained in the uterus (fig. 7.13). Retention of all or part of the placenta can lead to uterine infection, toxemia of the mare, and laminitis.

Dystocia (Difficult Delivery)

Miniature horse mares seem to be at a greater risk for **dystocia** than full-size mares. This is most likely related to their small size. Also, Miniature horse foals have a prominent dome on their forehead that can make positioning in the birth canal difficult (fig. 7.14). Delivery of a dwarf often results in a dystocia due to the abnormally large head seen in these foals.

It is critical that the person monitoring the delivery be trained to the signs of a problem with the delivery. Also, the veterinarian should be given warning when a mare is close to foaling. At that time, the veterinarian can outline his parameters for when he wants to be called during a delivery. For instance, a veterinarian that is located far from the breeding establishment may want to be notified as soon as the mare breaks water so that he has plenty of time to reach the farm if a problem develops. In other cases, especially when the veterinarian is familiar with the abilities of the foal-watch personnel, he may want to be called only when there is evidence that a problem is developing. Establishing a back-up veterinarian is advisable in case the primary veterinarian is occupied with another emergency at the same time as a dystocia.

It is also important to be prepared for the possibility of a severe dystocia where surgical intervention is necessary. The owner and veterinarian should discuss where the mare would be taken and when she should be transported if such a situation should arise. Some veterinarians prefer the mare be transported to the clinic at the first signs of a problem with the delivery while others will first attempt to correct the problem at the farm.

One valuable evaluation that can easily be taught to owners and foaling personnel is to determine the position of the foal. When the amniotic sac becomes visible, the sac can be broken and a clean, well-lubricated hand inserted to evaluate the position of the foal's feet and head. Ideally, in Miniature horses, the person with the smallest hands should be chosen for this procedure. The insertion of the hand should be done gently, and pushing against a mare's contraction is not recommended as it could cause injury to the mare's vagina. Insertion of the hand past the birth canal is also not recommended for fear of injury to the mare.

The following are indications that there may be a problem with the delivery and a veterinarian should be notified immediately:

- The mare has had several strong contractions and the amniotic sac has not appeared.
- The mare has been in Stage II labor for approaching an hour and the foal still has not been born. Even if the foal is partially out, failure to complete the delivery in this time period may be an indication of a problem with the positioning of the foal.
- Examination of the foal in the birth canal reveals that it is not positioned properly. Remember that the bottom of the front feet should be pointing downward, and one foot should be slightly behind the other with the head resting on top of, or to the side of the legs at the level of the carpi.
- Severe bulging of the rectum during delivery. This may indicate that the foal's foot is directed against the rectal wall, which could result in tearing of the rectum. Gently inserting a hand and re-directing the foot into a downward position will often prevent such an injury.
- The appearance of a red, velvety membrane at the vulva is called a red-bag delivery and is an indication that the placenta has separated off the wall of the uterus prematurely and the oxygen supply to the foal has been compromised (fig. 7.15). The membrane should be torn or cut and every attempt made to extract the foal as soon as possible.

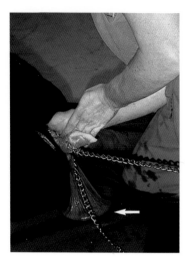

7.15 A red-bag delivery. The placenta (see arrow) has separated from the uterine wall prematurely. The mare was placed under anesthesia to facilitate rapid extraction of the foal. Chains are being used around the foal's legs for additional traction when pulling.

Walking the mare while waiting for the veterinarian's arrival will minimize her contractions. This is important in order to prevent a worsening of the problem. The mare's tail should be wrapped and the vulva and surrounding area cleaned in preparation for the veterinarian's arrival. The exception to this is in cases of a red-bag delivery where the foal should be extracted as soon as possible.

A clean, roomy area should be available for the veterinarian to work. This may be the foaling stall, but another area should be used if the foaling stall is too small to allow the mare to lie down and still give the veterinarian room to lay behind her and manipulate the foal.

Once the veterinarian evaluates the mare and position of the foal, he will make a decision as how best to deliver a live foal without undue injury to the mare. Sometimes this is just a simple manipulation, such as repositioning a front leg that has become locked at the elbow. In cases where the malpositioning is more severe and the mare is straining against the veterinarian, an epidural or general anesthesia may be used. If extraction of the foal is still unsuccessful, a cesarean section may be recommended. It is a good idea to prepare to transport a mare as soon as the dystocia is recognized. The truck and trailer can be readied while waiting for the veterinarian to arrive.

7.16 A dystocia in a Miniature horse mare. The mare's rear end is being lifted off the ground to shift the foal out of the birth canal into the uterus where there is more room for manipulation. The mare is also being prepped for a cesarean section in the event that the foal cannot be extracted vaginally.

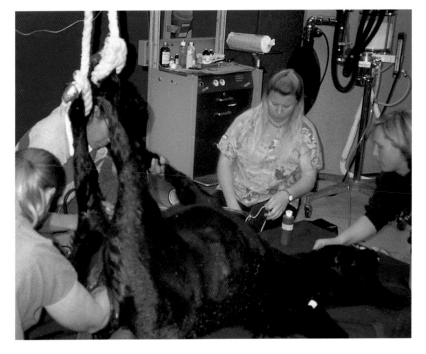

Another structure that I have found invaluable in cases of Miniature horse dystocias is a strong beam over the foaling stall or work area. The beam and supporting structures should be sturdy enough to support the weight of the mare. If attempts to correct a malpositioned foal in an awake mare are not successful, the mare is placed under anesthesia. Hobbles are placed around the back pasterns (after bandaging them for protection) and a rope is then attached to the hobbles and tossed over the beam. One strong person or two average people take hold of the rope and pull, lifting the mare's rear end off the ground (fig. 7.16). This shifts the foal out of the birth canal and into the uterus where additional extensive manipulations can be performed to reposition it.

In rare instances, the foal cannot be delivered vaginally because it is deformed or severely contracted. Examples of deformities that prevent vaginal delivery include misshapen legs, a neck that is fixed in a bent position, and an overly large or misshapen head. If the legs are fixed in a flexed position due to severe contracture, the foal will not fit through the birth canal.

When this situation arises, or examination by the veterinarian determines that the foal is dead, there are two options for extracting the foal—cesarean section or **fetotomy**. Fetotomy is a procedure where the foal's extremities are removed in order to allow it to fit through the birth canal.

While fetotomies are used successfully in full-sized mares, I have seen several ponies and Miniature horse mares whose cervix and vagina has been damaged by this procedure, rendering them unable to carry a foal again. For this reason, cesarean section is preferable to fetotomy unless a surgical facility is not available.

Postparturient Period

Most mares recover quite quickly after parturition and become focused on their foals. Minor periods of discomfort are normal for several days as the uterus begins to contract. Passage of bloodstained fluid from the vagina during this time period is also normal. Some mares are slow to defecate after foaling. This may be due to discomfort experienced when they push to pass the feces.

A veterinarian should examine the mare for any injuries that might have occurred during foaling. Usually this consists of a cursory exam of the vagina and vulva, but a more thorough exam is warranted if the mare had a difficult delivery. Some possible injuries include tearing of the cervix, lacerations of the vagina or vulva, or tearing the rectal wall or anus. Bruising of the vagina and vulva is normal.

It is a good idea to periodically check the mare's udder for several days. It should be examined both before and after the foal nurses. If the udder is small and dry before nursing, the mare may not be producing enough milk to support the foal. Another sign that the mare may not be producing enough milk is if the foal spends an inordinate amount of time at the udder trying to get enough to eat. If the udder is very full after nursing, the foal may not be eating adequately and should be observed closely for any other abnormalities. Some mares are prolific milk producers and always seem to have a full udder. Tenderness or swelling of one mammary gland may be an indication of infection and should be examined by a veterinarian.

A veterinarian should be contacted if any of the following signs are seen in the mare:

- Unwillingness to eat.
- Failure to pass feces within 24 hours after foaling.
- Signs of colic (see *Colic,* Chapter Four).
- Change in vaginal discharge from blood tinged to thick, white, or malodorous discharge.
- Unwillingness to allow the foal to nurse.

7.17 The foal should begin
to search for the udder soon
after standing. This youngster
has found the udder even
though his sense of balance is
still poorly developed. (Photo
courtesy of Vickie Swaroski).

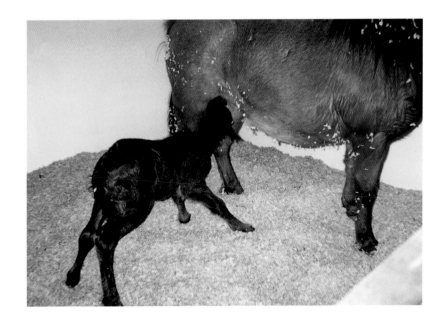

Hypocalcemia (Eclampsia, Lactation Tetany)

Hypocalcemia is a rare disorder of horses that is caused by low blood levels
of calcium. Miniature horse mares seem to be more at risk for this condition
compared to full-sized mares.

Calcium plays a vital role in muscle function, including cardiac muscle.
When blood levels are low, the horse will demonstrate muscle stiffness,
stilted gait, muscle twitches, weakness, anxiety, sweating, increased heart
rate, and irregular heart rhythms. A classic sign of hypocalcemia is a condition called thumps or synchronous diaphragmatic flutter where the
diaphragm contracts every time the heart beats (similar to hiccups in time
with the heart). If left untreated, hypocalcemia can progress to convulsions,
coma, and death.

CAUSES

Loss of calcium into the milk is the main cause of hypocalcemia in mares. In
most cases, a stressful event seems to initiate the disorder. For example,
hypocalcemia can occur secondary to transportation, surgery, vaccination,
breeding, or weaning. How stress predisposes a mare to hypocalcemia is
unknown.

DIAGNOSIS

Hypocalcemia should be suspected in any late-term pregnant mare or lactating mare that is exhibiting signs of muscle weakness or stiffness, or has an

abnormal cardiac rhythm. Thumps are diagnostic for hypocalcemia. Measurement of calcium levels in the blood not only provide the diagnosis of hypocalcemia, it provides a quantitative measure of the severity of the disorder.

TREATMENT

Treatment consists of the intravenous administration of calcium. The calcium is administered as a 20 percent solution of calcium gluconate and must be given slowly as rapid administration can affect the normal activity of the heart. Repeated treatments may be necessary. Whenever possible, the stress that initiated the event should be eliminated to prevent a relapse.

PROGNOSIS

In general, the prognosis for successful treatment of hypocalcemia is good. However, the disorder can be fatal if it is not correctly diagnosed and calcium administered.

The Foal

Post-Foaling Care

The umbilical cord usually breaks when the mare stands after foaling. Once the cord breaks, the umbilical stump (naval) should be dipped or painted with betadine or chlorhexidine solution. Care should be taken to avoid getting these solutions on the foal's skin as it may irritate or blister it. This treatment should be repeated four or five times during the first twenty-four hours. The foal should also be given a tetanus vaccine if the mare was not vaccinated within six weeks of foaling.

Shortly after being born, the foal will begin to make attempts to stand. Most foals will stand within an hour of being born. Miniature horse foals are especially quick to get to their feet, possibly because of their low center of gravity. I have seen Miniature horse foals stand within fifteen minutes of birth. If the foal does not begin making attempts to stand within the first fifteen minutes or has not stood within the hour, a veterinarian should be notified. Once the foal is standing, its legs can be evaluated for abnormalities such as contractures, laxities, or angular limb deformities (ALDs) that may need veterinary attention (see *Abnormalities of Growth*, p. 15).

After standing, the foal will begin to search for the teat and should nurse within two hours of being born (fig. 7.17). The foal may become weak if it does not eat in that two-hour time period. If the mare is moving about, inhibiting the foal's ability to find the udder, a handler can halter her and

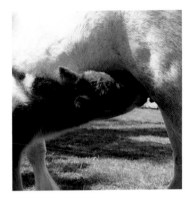

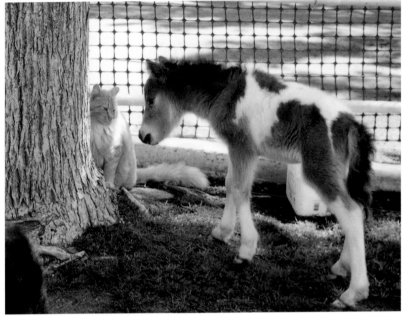

7.18 A–C A normal, healthy foal will be curious of its surroundings, nurse frequently, and sleep soundly.

hold her still. Some movement of the mare is normal and seems to be an important tool in teaching the foal to follow the mare. However, if the foal has been chasing the mare for more than an hour, intervention is warranted. It is important that all interactions with the mare and foal be done as quietly and calmly as possible. The veterinarian should be contacted if the foal does not nurse within the first two hours.

Meconium is the fecal material that forms while the foal is still in the uterus. It has a black, tarry appearance. The meconium can become impacted in the large colon or rectum. The most common sign of a meconium impaction is the foal straining to defecate, but signs of colic may be seen in the more severe cases. Veterinary care should be sought any time a foal is seen straining to defecate.

Many breeders routinely administer an enema to a newborn foal to prevent meconium impaction. Over-the-counter pediatric enemas work well in Miniature horse foals. The foal should be restrained and the enema inserted gently to minimize the chance of injury to the rectum. Passage of softer, brown feces signals that all the meconium has passed and the foal is passing fecal material produced since birth (milk feces).

The foal should be observed for urination during the first two to three days. In rare instances, a foal's bladder can rupture during the birthing process. This is more common in male foals; the narrow diameter of their urethra allows a greater pressure buildup in the bladder. The best time to

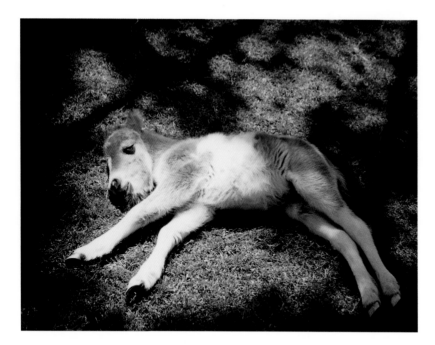

watch for urination is after the foal gets up from a nap. It will usually nurse, then urinate shortly after nursing. Signs of a ruptured bladder are straining to urinate, colic, bloated abdomen, weakness, and loss of appetite.

Blood should be drawn from the foal when it is between sixteen and twenty-four hours old. The blood level of IgG, the type of antibody supplied by the mare's colostrum, is measured to determine if the foal received adequate colostrum to be protected from infection. The veterinarian can also perform a complete physical of the foal and mare as well as examine the placenta at the time the blood is drawn.

Indications of Disease

A healthy foal is bright, alert, and full of energy. It will nurse at least once every hour. It is curious of its surroundings and between nursing and playing, will sleep soundly (figs. 7.18 A–C).

The following are signs of illness or disease in a foal and are indicators that veterinary attention should be obtained.

- The foal does not stand within one hour of birth or nurse within two hours of birth.
- The foal does not search for the udder or bond with the mare.

- Straining to urinate or defecate.
- Depression or loss of appetite (the foal is not seen nursing or the mare's udder is constantly full).
- Frequent rolling from side to side or laying on its back when sleeping.
- Signs of colic.
- Lameness.
- Swelling of, or discharge from the umbilicus.
- Urinating out of the umbilicus.
- Swelling in the inguinal (groin) area.
- Fever (see *Normal Physical Parameters*, Appendix A).
- Failure to gain weight.
- Coughing.
- Milk coming from its nose (see *Cleft Palate*, p. 44).
- Difficulty breathing or abnormal respiratory noise (see Chapter Two).
- Squinting or holding its eyes closed.

In general, Miniature horse foals have few medical problems. However, minor problems can easily become life threatening if early treatment is not initiated.

Summary

There are few differences between Miniature horses and full-sized horses in the area of reproduction. With respect to stallion management, the most important differences involve normal parameters for semen, the use of appropriate equipment for semen collection, and knowing the rules established by the AMHA with respect to artificial insemination.

While the general principles of mare management in Miniature horses are the same as full-sized horses, the small size of the Miniature horse mare does present a bit of a challenge when evaluating the ovaries and in pregnancy detection. Also, because of a greater tendency to late-term abortion and dystocia, pregnant Miniature horse mares should be monitored closely throughout the last trimester of their pregnancy and should always be attended during delivery.

The care of Miniature horse foals is the same as for other breeds. Close observation during the first several days after birth insures that any abnormality will be identified early in the course of the disease. Early treatment of disease in foals is critical as they can become gravely ill in a relatively short period of time.

CHAPTER 8

Nutrition

By Stephen Duren, Ph.D.

YOU CAN OMIT a lot of the things you do to and for your horse. You can almost certainly forget to buy the spray that helps make your horse's coat shine. You can occasionally forget to clean out his feet. You can be a couple of weeks late on deworming, or wait another week before calling your farrier to trim his feet. However, you cannot neglect feeding your horse. For its body to work properly, your horse needs to eat properly.

It should come as no surprise, if you have a performance horse you need to feed it properly so it performs to its capabilities. Likewise, pregnant mares and young horses need to be fed appropriately so that sound foals are produced and eventually grow to be healthy adults. Most people who own Miniature horses have a strong desire to properly feed their animals. Many horse owners, however, get lost in the vast array of nutrition choices and end up with poor feeding programs. Feeding the Miniature horse, as well as any other type of horse, does not need to be difficult. The key to proper feeding is to understand the basics and to keep your nutritional goals in mind.

The Basics

What's in Feed?

From oats to apples, all feeds contain nutrients. The only difference among feedstuffs is the amount of nutrients each offers. Because all feeds provide nutrients, it is no longer appropriate to label feeds as "good" or "bad." Feeds should be discussed by their nutrient content. This allows horse owners to make reasonable choices about what they are going to feed their horse and why. The nutrients contained in feed are energy, protein, vitamins, minerals, and water.

Energy

Energy runs the chemical reactions in the body, supplies the fuel that stimulates the heart to beat and muscles to contract, fosters fetal development in mares, and supports the milk production that initiates and promotes growth in young horses. For most horses, 80–90 percent of the feed consumed is used to satisfy energy requirements. Thus, the main focus of any diet is energy. The energy content of a feed is measured in units called calories. Energy is not an actual nutrient per se. Instead, energy results from the digestion of carbohydrates, proteins, and fats.

In plant-eating animals such as horses, carbohydrates are the primary source of energy. Approximately 75 percent of all plant material is made up of carbohydrates. Different types of carbohydrates are found in horse feed, and the horse is able to digest and use these assorted carbohydrates to varying degrees.

Carbohydrates can be divided into two broad categories, structural and nonstructural. Structural carbohydrates are known as plant fiber and act as the skeleton of the plant. These are tough, rigid compounds, so tough, in fact, that no mammalian digestive system produces chemicals or enzymes that can break them down. However, horses are able to make use of plant fiber because of bacteria that live in their digestive tracts. About 50 percent of the plant fiber taken in by horses is digestible, and the rest is simply passed out in the manure. Conversely, nonstructural carbohydrates are composed of sugars, the most common being starch. Grain is rich in starch. On average, 90 percent of nonstructural carbohydrates are digestible by horses.

Fat is another source of energy for horses. On a pound for pound basis, fat provides approximately three times as much energy as oats and two and one-half times as much energy as corn. Natural feedstuffs given to horses, such as hay and simple grains, contain small amounts of fat. The most common sources of fat given to horses are vegetable oils (corn oil and soybean oil, for example) and high-fat stabilized rice bran.

Finally, protein fed in excess of requirements can be used for energy. The digestion of protein for energy production is inefficient and produces nitrogen as a by-product. Nitrogen must be excreted in the urine. Therefore, protein is thought of as "metabolically expensive." Not only does it tax metabolism, but protein is the most expensive ingredient in a ration, so the use of it as an energy source is unwise.

Protein

Protein is a major component of hair, hoof, skin, muscle, blood cells, enzymes, and hormones. Once water and fat are removed, 80 percent of the body is composed of protein. Protein is used to build new tissues and repair damaged ones. Proteins are composed of amino acids. Individual amino acids are chemically bound in various arrangements to assimilate the many proteins of the body. Think of the individual amino acids as letters in the alphabet and the complete proteins as the words created by those letters.

Most horse owners are concerned about the proper amount of protein in the feed. The protein content of feed is listed on the feed tag. The amount of protein required in the diet depends on the requirement of an individual horse, the quality of protein being fed, and the amount of feed the horse is eating. Given that many horse owners are concerned about protein levels, the following levels of protein in the total diet provide an appropriate starting point:

Mature (Maintenance)	8–10%
Mature (Training)	10–12%
Pregnant Mares	11–12%
Lactating Mares	13–14%
Weanlings	14.5–16%
Yearlings	13–14%

Vitamins

Vitamins are essential for all metabolic functions within a horse. Horsemen are often concerned about vitamin levels in feeds. Much of this concern is unwarranted, however, because horses can create within their body sufficient quantities of all vitamins except vitamins A and E.

Vitamins are divided into two classes, fat-soluble and water-soluble. Fat-soluble vitamins (A, D, E, and K) are stored in the fat reserves of the body. As such, caution is advised as oversupplementation with vitamins is possible, and toxicity or poisoning may occur, especially with vitamins A and D. Water-soluble vitamins, including the B-vitamins and vitamin C, are not stored in the body. Due to their solubility, oversupplementation of these vitamins is not considered a health risk.

Minerals

Minerals are inorganic substances that are needed by the horse for normal metabolic and biological activity. Unlike vitamins, minerals cannot be created by the horse, thus, they need to be supplied in the diet. Fortunately, most common feeds contain a variety of important minerals. The mineral content of feedstuffs varies depending on the soil in which the feed is grown. Therefore, it is customary to add minerals to commercial horse feeds.

Although minerals are needed by the horse, they should only be supplemented to correct for specific mineral deficiencies in a diet. Too much mineral supplementation is as detrimental as too little.

Minerals are often divided into two categories. Macrominerals are necessary in large amounts in the diet. Examples of macrominerals include calcium, phosphorus, magnesium, sodium, and chloride. Microminerals are required in micro or small amounts in the diet. Examples of microminerals include copper, zinc, selenium, and iodine.

Water

Water is the single most important nutrient in the diet. A horse can lose almost all of its body fat and over 50 percent of its body protein and still survive. However, a loss of only 10 percent of the its water reservoir can be devastating to the health of a horse. Water functions as a coolant, as a universal solvent for many of the chemical reactions in the body, and as a carrier of nutrients to and waste products away from the cells in the body. The water requirement of the horse varies based on environmental temperature, exercise or activity, lactation, and the type and amount of feed consumed. As a practical guideline, horses should have unlimited access to fresh, clean water.

In sum, horses must be supplied with sufficient quantities of energy, protein, vitamins, minerals, and water. Learning how a horse utilizes the nutrients in feed is the next step in understanding basic horse nutrition.

Utilizing Feed—The Digestive System

The digestive tract of the horse is divided into two distinct areas based on the type of digestion that occurs. The front portion of the digestive system, sometimes called the foregut, features enzymatic digestion, and the hindgut is designed for bacterial fermentation.

The horse begins the digestive process by taking feed into the mouth and chewing. For this process to be efficient, the horse needs a sound, functional mouth. Chewing and the presence of food in the mouth stimulate the flow of saliva, which lubricates the food and enables ease of swallowing. Food passes from the mouth, travels down the esophagus, and lands in the stomach. The stomach of an adult horse is very small compared to its body size, thus limiting meal size. In the stomach, the digestive process continues as acid mixes with the feed. From the stomach, food passes into the small intestine, the main site of enzymatic digestion and absorption.

Feed not digested in the stomach and small intestine moves into the hindgut for fermentation by microorganisms. The hindgut consists of the cecum and colon (see *Anatomy of the Gastrointestinal Tract*, p. 59). Billions of bacteria and protozoa work together in the hindgut to break down plant fiber. The intestinal microorganisms produce energy-yielding compounds called volatile fatty acids, as well as amino acids and B-vitamins. In addition, the hindgut is responsible for the absorption of water and electrolytes from the diet. Undigested material advances into the rectum and is passed as manure. The entire digestive process takes 24 to 72 hours.

Lessons Learned from the Digestive System
The anatomy of the digestive system provides several clues on how to properly feed horses. Mistakes made in feeding horses can result in serious health issues, including colic and laminitis. First, the digestive system contains a simple stomach. The size of the stomach reveals that horses are best suited to small, frequent meals rather than large meals. Second, digestion should be continuous. In the absence of food, the stomach accumulates acid and causes the formation of ulcers, which may adversely affect growth or performance. Horses perform optimally if they have hay or pasture in front of them at all times.

The grain (starch) portion of the diet is intended to be digested in the small intestine. If too much grain is fed in a single meal or accidental overfeeding occurs, the small intestine is unable to digest all of the starch it is presented. The excess starch spills into the hindgut, where bacterial fermentation occurs. This causes a rapid increase in gut acidity and the potential for laminitis increases greatly (see *Laminitis*, p. 11). The grain portion of the diet should be limited such that a grain meal is no more than 1.25 pounds of grain per 250 pounds of body weight.

Finally, roughly 65 percent of the digestive capacity of the gastrointestinal system is dedicated to the digestion of plant fiber. This indicates that forage (such as hay or pasture) should be the main ingredient in any diet. Forage helps horses feel full and provides "chewing satisfaction." A constant source of fiber is essential for the health of bacteria in the hindgut. Plus, a certain amount of bulk in the diet is needed to sustain normal digestive function. Horses deprived of adequate fiber usually let their owners know by seeking out alternative fiber sources, including wood fences, stall fronts, and trees.

Feed Choices

The selection of feedstuffs suitable for horses is tremendous. To understand the different feeding options, it is helpful to classify feeds according to their nutrient profile. When grouped by nutrient content, feed choices are reduced to forage, unfortified grains, fortified grain concentrates, and supplements.

Forage

The most common forages fed to horses include pasture, baled hay, hay cubes, hay pellets, and beet pulp.

Pasture

Pasture is the most natural forage for horses. High-quality pasture can provide horses with every essential nutrient except water. In addition, pasture is relatively inexpensive. To be considered high quality, pasture must have an adequate stand of nutritious plant life, few weeds, and no poisonous plants (see Appendix B). Advice on which grasses to plant in a certain geographical region can be obtained by consulting extension personnel at a university, a horse nutritionist, or a veterinarian. A pasture should also be large enough to prevent horses from overgrazing and damaging the plants. Because pasture is not something weighed and measured accurately prior to feeding, as in the case of hay or grain, intake must be controlled by limiting grazing time. If horses are becoming overweight on pasture, the amount of time they are allowed to graze should be reduced.

Hay

Hay is made from green plants that are mowed in mid growth, preserved by drying, and stored to be fed at a later date. Just about any type of plant can be made into hay, although not all hays are equally nutritious for the horse. Top-quality hay begins with nutritious plants. Plants must be harvested at the proper stage of maturity to maximize nutrient content. If plants are allowed to become too mature (tall and coarse), hay made from them resembles baled sticks. Once the plants are cut, they must be allowed to dry, so they will not spoil while in storage.

The value of high-quality hay cannot be overemphasized. Moldy hay is a potential source of medical problems. Dusty hay is a source of irritation to the respiratory tract and has been implicated as a cause of airway problems. Rodents, rabbits, and any other small animals that get caught up in the hay-baling equipment are a potential source of botulism. A simple rule of thumb works well when feeding hay—if the hay is suspect, do not feed it.

Hays generally can be divided into two types. Legume hays such as alfalfa and clover have microorganisms associated with their root system. These microorganisms are able to use the nitrogen in the air and soil to produce protein. Grass hays such as timothy and orchard grass or cereal grain hays such as oat contain lower protein, less energy, less calcium, fewer vitamins, and more fiber than legume hays. Legume, grass, and cereal grain hays are all perfectly acceptable for horses, as long as the nutrient content of the entire diet is properly balanced.

Hay Pellets and Hay Cubes

Hay pellets and hay cubes are other forms of forage suitable for horses. Hay is condensed into pellets or cubes by first chopping it into small pieces. Steam is then added to the chopped hay, and it is forced through a pellet or cube die so the pieces of chopped hay bind to one another. Hay pellets and cubes are well accepted by horses once they become familiar with eating little bricks of hay instead of conventional long-stem hay. On the plus side, hay pellets and cubes are easy to store and measure and eaten with virtually no waste. Horses consume the same weight of cubes or pellets as long-stem hay. For instance, if a Miniature horse typically is offered five pounds of hay, it would be given five pounds of pellets or cubes. There is no difference in digestibility between baled hay, cubed hay, or pelleted hay.

Beet Pulp

Beet pulp is the fibrous by product of the extraction of table sugar from sugar beets. It is a high-energy fiber alternative, which is gaining in popularity with Miniature horse owners and trainers as it provides dietary fiber without producing the hay belly caused by feeding hay as the sole fiber source.

Beet pulp comes either shredded or pelleted and can be fed wet or dry. Most horses find it to be palatable, and because it is less fibrous than hay, is more easily chewed and digested. Its energy is slowly released after microbial fermentation in the cecum and colon, unlike the carbohydrates in grain that are quickly absorbed in the small intestine. Therefore, beet pulp can be used to add calories to a horse's diet without increasing the risk of colic or laminitis. As a result, beet pulp is an excellent feed for thin horses, debilitated horses, and horses that have difficulty chewing because of dental abnormalities.

There are several facts about beet pulp that should be considered before introducing it as a forage alternative. Firstly, eating beet pulp does not satisfy a horse's innate urge to graze. Horses that receive only beet pulp as their fiber source will frequently resort to eating bedding, wood fences, or stalls in an effort to satisfy this urge. Therefore, incorporating beet pulp into a diet with hay is a better approach in most cases than feeding beet pulp alone.

Beet pulp is very high in calcium. Combining it with alfalfa, also very high in calcium, may lead to an imbalance in the calcium:phosphorus ratio in the diet which is important for normal bone and muscle development. Combining it with grass hay, which is typically low in calcium, is a better choice.

Finally, beet pulp is very high in energy. It provides more calories than any other forage source—as much as 25 percent more than grass hay. Careful observation for weight gain is important when feeding beet pulp to Miniature horses that tend toward obesity.

Unfortified Grain

Unfortified grain is the seed head of a plant that is harvested from the field and dried to a suitable moisture content for storage. Such grains include oats, corn, barley, wheat, and milo. These grains are considered unfortified because they do not have protein, vitamins, or minerals added to enhance their nutritive value.

Unfortified grain can be further subdivided into whole grains and processed grains. Unfortunately, with the single exception of oats, whole grains are not ideal for horses because they have a hard outer hull that protects the starch portion of the grain. Consequently, it is difficult for the horse to digest most whole grains in the small intestine. Grain should be mechanically processed prior to feeding to horses. There are many different ways to process grain, such as cracking, crimping, flaking, grinding, and rolling. These processing methods break the grain kernel and increase the surface area for digestion.

Fortified Concentrates

Fortified concentrates are most often fed to horses. These products often include several processed grains and a protein, vitamin, and mineral supplement package. The supplementation is added by the feed manufacturer and typically includes both fat- and water-soluble vitamins, along with macro- and microminerals.

Fortified grain concentrates can be purchased in several different physical forms, depending on processing preference. Examples of the different physical forms available include textured feeds, pellets, extruded nuggets, and combinations of the three forms. Textured feeds contain a blend of processed (usually cracked or crimped) grain with a light coating of molasses and occasionally vegetable oil. The result is a moist, sticky mix often called "sweet feed." Pelleted grain concentrates contain ground grains along with supplemental protein, vitamins, and minerals. The ground materials are mixed together, conditioned with steam, and forced into a pellet-sized die. Extruded products also contain ground grain along with supplemental protein, vitamins, and minerals. The mixture is exposed to extreme heat and pressure, which actually changes the physical nature of the grain, so it can be formed into different shapes.

Supplements

By definition, a supplement is provided "to complete something, to make up for a deficiency, or to extend and strengthen the whole." Supplements are advertised to cure or help with most horse problems, including rough hair coat, cracked hooves, hyperactivity, sweat loss, anemia, and the list goes on. Supplements are often given in an effort to "improve" the horse. This means that the supplement is given because the owner wants the horse to be somehow better or different than it actually is. The reality with nutrient supplementation is that extra amounts of a nutrient will not supercharge performance if there is not a preexisting deficiency. In other words, giving a blood-building supplement with massive amounts of iron will not make the blood superior if the horse was not deficient in iron originally.

On the other hand, many supplements can be helpful if they are part of a balanced feeding program. Before adding any supplement, care should be taken to make sure a horse actually needs the nutrients provided in the supplement. If fed a fortified concentrate at the recommended level, a horse probably does not require a supplement. It should be noted that certain vitamins and minerals, including vitamin A, vitamin D, selenium, and iodine, can be toxic if overfed to horses.

The Ground Rules

In many ways, feeding a horse is much like using a roadmap. Different roads can lead to the same destination. Likewise, many different feeding choices can result in a balanced diet. When driving there are certain rules of the road that must be followed, such as stopping at red lights and obeying the speed limit. In regard to feeding horses, following certain rules will increase the likelihood of achieving a balanced diet. Before delving into the ground rules of feeding horses, there are two basic principles that must be understood.

First, to feed horses properly caretakers must have a realistic idea of how much the horse weighs. This is important because the nutrient requirements, which ultimately determine how much is fed, are based on body weight. Calculating weight can be accomplished by several means. A scale is by far the most accurate means of determining weight. Unfortunately, most people do not own scales to accommodate even a Miniature horse. Scales large enough to weigh a Miniature horse may be found at grain elevators or veterinary clinics.

The second means of determining weight is to eyeball the horse. Achieving accurate weight assessment using this method is difficult unless the evaluator is experienced. A study done by Kentucky Equine Research found that most owners of Miniature horses tend to misjudge weight by over 20 percent. Approximately 50 percent of Miniature horse owners underestimated the weight of their horses by an average of 36 pounds, and 48 percent of owners overestimated the weight of their horses by an average of 54 pounds. The average body weight for the Miniature horses in that study was 213 pounds.

The third method used to determine body weight is a weight tape. Weight tapes can be obtained from a variety of sources, including feed stores and horse catalogs. Most weight tapes are not accurate on Miniature horses.

A fourth way to determine body weight uses body measurements and a simple formula. This is accomplished by measuring the length of the horse from the point of the shoulder to the point of the buttocks and by measuring the distance around the girth at the withers. These numbers are then put into the following equation to determine body weight:

BW (pounds) equals 9.36 x girth (inches) + 5.01 x body length (inches) minus 348.53 (fig. 8.1).

Once body weight is determined, feed must be weighed. Vague measurement units such as "flakes" and "coffee cans" are unsuitable when properly evaluating a ration. If the elements of a diet are weighed and accurately measured using any type of scale, the horse will be more likely to receive what it actually needs.

Feeding horses has certain steadfast rules. If these rules are followed, many nutritional problems can be avoided. Fortunately, there are just a few rules to remember:

1. The majority of the diet must be composed of forage. At least 50 percent of what is fed to a horse has to consist of either pasture, hay, hay cubes, hay pellets, or beet pulp. The fiber in forage is absolutely necessary in order to maintain proper gut function.
2. Horses should always have unlimited access to clean, fresh water.
3. Horses should always be fed high-quality feed. Low-grade feed may lack virtually every nutrient that a feed is supposed to provide.

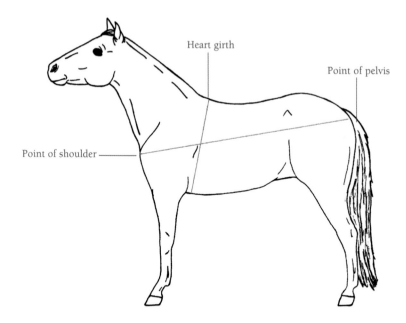

8.1 A Miniature horse's body weight can be calculated from measurements of body length (red line) and heart girth (green line). See text for the equation.

Feed contaminated with mold, dust, and foreign material should be discarded. Because a horse has a one-way digestive tract, it is unable to eliminate disagreeable feed by vomiting.

4. Monitor energy intake. Energy is the only dietary factor that caretakers can visually assess. If a horse takes in too much energy (eats too much feed), it becomes overweight. If a horse consumes too little dietary energy, he becomes underweight. Whether a horse is too fat or too thin, the blame likely should be assigned to the caretaker.

5. If grain is fed, never feed more than 1.25 pounds of grain per 250 pounds of horse in a single feeding. This would calculate to no more than 1.5 pounds of grain per meal for a 300-pound horse. Grain meals should be kept small to avoid undigested starch (grain) reaching the hindgut and undergoing dangerous fermentation.

6. Feed regularly from day to day and at least twice a day.

7. Dietary changes should be done slowly over a period of two to three weeks. This will help avoid digestive upset or colic.

Feeding the Horse at Maintenance

To determine a proper diet for any horse, a logical starting point must be established. That starting point does not take into account whether a horse is expected to gain weight, to exercise regularly, or to nurse a foal, activities that require extra nutrients. The amount of feed that must be provided to a horse to keep it alive, without losing weight, is a reasonable beginning place. This is called feeding for maintenance, and such a program is well suited for mature, idle geldings, barren mares, and breeding stallions in the off-season.

Maintaining a horse's weight with a diet consisting of high-quality forage, water, salt, and possibly a trace mineral supplement (depending on the nutrient content of the forage) is feasible. As a minimum, a horse will need 1.5 percent of its body weight per day in forage to maintain weight. For example, if a Miniature horse weighs 250 pounds, it will need a minimum of 3.75 pounds of hay.

Horses can certainly eat more than 1.5 percent of their body weight in forage if permitted. Some horses can easily consume 3 percent of their body weight in forage on a given day. If a horse maintains its weight on 1.5 percent of its body weight in forage per day, an increase in the amount of hay provided is unnecessary. On the other hand, if a horse loses condition on this amount of hay, slowly increasing the amount of hay given will allow it to gain weight until a maintenance allotment can be calculated. Most horses at maintenance will not require grain, or perhaps only small amounts of grain, to maintain condition if high-quality forage is fed. In addition to hay and possibly grain, the horse fed for maintenance should have unlimited access to water and salt.

After calculating how much a horse weighs and how much to feed it, an idea of how much it should weigh should be considered. In other words, is the horse in optimum condition? Is it obese or ribby? Table 2 on page 131 is a "condition-score" chart adapted from D.R. Henneke, first published in *Equine Veterinary Journal* in 1983.[28]

Feeding the Overweight Horse

Remember, if a horse is fat, it is the fault of its caretaker. After all, horses love to eat, and they can only eat what is offered to them. If a horse is overweight, a combination of feed restriction and exercise will facilitate weight loss. Care should be taken not to reduce forage intake below 1 percent of body weight. If forage is restricted beyond this level, the digestive system will not function properly. Switching the overweight horse to a lower-energy hay (from alfalfa hay to grass hay, for example) will reduce calorie intake. Exercise should begin gradually and increase in intensity. Weight loss will take time.

28 Henneke, DR. Relationship between condition score, physical measurements and body fat percentage in mares. *Eq Vet Journal* 1983; 15:371

1	POOR	Extremely emaciated; back bones, ribs, tailhead, and hip bones project prominently; bone structure of withers, shoulders, and neck easily noticeable; no fatty tissue can be felt.
2	VERY THIN	Emaciated; slight fat covering over base of back bones; vertebrae feel rounded; back bones, ribs, tailhead, and hip bones prominent; withers, shoulders, and neck structures are faintly discernible.
3	THIN	Fat buildup about halfway on back bones; slight fat cover over ribs, back bones easily felt; tailhead prominent but individual vertebrae cannot be identified visually; hip bones rounded but easily seen; withers, neck, and shoulder accentuated.
4	MODERATELY THIN	Slight ridge along back; faint outline of the ribs discernible; tailhead prominence depends on conformation, fat can be felt around it; hip bones not discernible; withers, shoulders, and neck not obviously thin.
5	MODERATE	Back is flat (no crease or ridge); ribs not visually distinguishable but easily felt; fat around tailhead beginning to feel spongy; withers appear rounded over back bones; shoulders and neck blend smoothly into body.
6	MODERATELY FLESHY	May have slight crease down back; fat over ribs is spongy; fat around tailhead soft; fat beginning to be deposited along the side of withers, behind shoulders, and along neck.
7	FLESHY	May have crease down back; individual ribs can be felt but noticeable filling between ribs with fat; fat around tailhead soft; fat deposited along withers, behind shoulders, and along neck.
8	FAT	Crease down back; difficult to feel ribs; fat around tailhead very soft; area along withers filled with fat; areas behind shoulders filled with fat; noticeable thickening of neck; fat deposited along inner thighs.
9	EXTREMELY FAT	Obvious crease down back, patchy fat over ribs; bulging fat around tailhead, along withers, behind shoulders, and along neck; fat along inner thighs may rub together; flank filled with fat.

Table 2 A "condition-score" chart.

Feeding the Underweight Horse

A thin horse presents unique challenges. Any number of factors can result in a horse becoming underweight, but as a practical matter, the most common causes of thinness are feed-related. Generally, a horse is too thin because its feed is of such poor quality that it is impossible for it to satisfy nutritional requirements of the horse. Another possible reason for an underweight horse is a general lack of feed. Granted, horses may have a parasite infestation, dental problem, or liver ailment that contributes to thinness, but feed quality or quantity is usually the culprit.

Another possible factor is "pecking order," a well-defined layer of dominance within a herd. The horses on the bottom of the pecking order will be chased away from feed by more domineering members of the herd and will often not get adequate opportunity to eat. Regrouping horses often solves this problem. Once the cause of thinness is identified, it may take months for the horse to regain weight. Drastic feed changes to accomplish rapid weight gain should be avoided due to the potential for digestive upset.

Feeding the Older Horse

A horse is considered "nutritionally old" when it can no longer eat its regular diet and maintain weight. As a horse ages, it loses some digestive efficiency and requires more feed to maintain condition. Some published reports target the nutrient requirements of aged horses to be approximately those of growing horses. Old horses need diets that consist of high-quality fiber and elevated protein and mineral levels. Care should be taken to ensure that proper dental care is maintained along with regular health care. To compensate for loss of teeth, hay products may need to be ground for older horses. Pelleted hay, cubed hay, or beet pulp soaked in water prior to feeding make a suitably rich fiber source for older horses. Additional calories can be provided in pelleted, fortified concentrates. These concentrates should contain additional fat to increase the energy density of the diet.

Feeding the Stallion

Stallions typically do not have any special nutrient requirements. Depending on the number of mares to be bred and the level of anxiety of the stallion, however, extra energy in the diet may be warranted. Breeding stallions may have energy requirements that are as much as 25 percent above what is needed for maintenance. Increased energy requirements can often be satisfied by providing more hay or by feeding a concentrate fortified with fat. Contrary to popular belief, breeding stallions do not benefit from megadoses of vitamins or minerals during the breeding season.

Feeding the Broodmare

During the first seven months of pregnancy, the mare does not have significantly elevated nutrient requirements above maintenance. At this time, the developing fetus is small and adds only slightly to the nutrient requirements of the mare. In early pregnancy, therefore, mares can be fed much like mature horses at maintenance.

During the last trimester (110 days) of pregnancy, the nutrient requirements of the mare and fetus increase drastically. Requirements for energy, protein, calcium, phosphorus, and vitamin A increase. Trying to get these additional nutrients into the pregnant mare is further complicated by the fact that as pregnancy progresses, the stomach of the mare may be crowded by the growing foal, decreasing her desire and ability to eat. This issue is often solved by feeding the mare more concentrated sources of nutrients. Feeding premium hay and well-fortified concentrates intended for broodmares will usually satisfy nutrient requirements. The diet for pregnant mares should contain a minimum of 50 percent forage. Grain concentrates can be fed at a rate of 0.5–1.0 percent of body weight.

The lactating mare has the highest nutrient requirements of any adult horse. Nutrients are being utilized for milk production and repair of tissues damaged during pregnancy. During the first three months of lactation, mares can easily consume 3 percent of their body weight per day in feed. This is roughly twice the amount of feed they would require in a maintenance situation. These mares should receive top-quality hay and likely will need to be supplemented with a vitamin- and mineral-fortified concentrate. A typical diet for a lactating mare would consist of free-choice hay and grain at a rate of 0.5–1.5 percent of body weight per day. The amount of grain should be adjusted depending on the body condition of the mare. Interestingly, the amount of vitamins and minerals consumed by the mare do not seem to significantly influence the nutrient composition of the milk. Instead, the amount of energy the mare receives determines the total amount of milk produced by the mare. Underfed mares will not produce adequate milk for a suckling.

Feeding the Growing Horse

Much discussion exists about the best way to feed a young horse. In reality, feeding a young horse is no different than feeding any other horse in that certain nutritional requirements must be met, and those needs can be fulfilled by a number of feed combinations. The most important nutritional factors to consider in growing horses are energy, protein, calcium, and phosphorus. Other minerals and vitamins are also important but not nearly as vital as the foregoing nutrients.

Energy is the dietary factor most associated with growth. As the amount of energy the foal receives increases, more calories are available to fuel growth. If too much energy is fed, foals will grow rapidly and may be prone to growth-related problems. Protein is often blamed for growth problems, but excessive protein has not been shown to be directly linked to abnormal growth. Growing foals require protein to develop both muscle and bone, and without adequate protein, growth will be slowed.

The two primary minerals to be concerned with in growing horses are calcium and phosphorus. These two minerals are critical because they make up a large proportion of the mineral content in the skeleton. Adequate amounts of calcium and phosphorus, in the correct ratio, must be provided. In the total diet (hay and grain), a ratio of two parts calcium to one part phosphorus (2:1), is considered ideal.

Feeding the young horse supplemental feed should begin at two to three months of age. At this time, the nutrient requirements of the foal begin to outpace the nutrients provided by milk. Foals should receive a fortified concentrate designed for growing horses. Commercial concentrates are very palatable and a wise choice for young horses. Remember, Miniature horses are approximately one-fifth to one-fourth the size of full-sized light horses; therefore, the amount of grain recommended on the feed bag should be reduced by that amount. Hay or pasture should be provided free choice.

Once the foals have reached approximately four months of age, they can be weaned at any time. Foals should be adapted to eating their own feed prior to weaning to minimize stress. The amount of grain concentrate should be gradually increased to maintain body condition. By the time the young horse is a late weanling, much of the skeletal growth has occurred and the growth rate will slow. The concentrate fed to yearlings usually contains lower levels of nutrients than those used for foals and weanlings. Again, making volume adjustments to the manufacturer's recommendations for concentrates works well. As with the foal and weanling, forage should be offered to yearlings on a free-choice basis.

Feeding the Performance Horse

Exercise makes unique demands on a horse. From a nutritional standpoint, the dietary factor most influenced by exercise is energy. Performance horses require energy to fuel muscle contraction, the very essence of exercise. To satisfy the increased energy demands of exercise, the horse will require more feed.

The foundation of the diet should always be high-quality forage. Performance horses are typically fed mixed alfalfa-grass or grass forage. Pure alfalfa is generally not fed because performance horses do not benefit from the large amount of protein it contains. For horses in light work, less than one hour per day, the energy requirements often can be satisfied by feeding more forage. Some horses performing the same amount of work will need small amounts of a vitamin- and mineral-fortified concentrate, approximately 0.5 percent of their body weight. As the intensity of exercise increases, feeding more hay will not satisfy energy requirements. Horses in heavy work simply cannot eat enough forage to maintain condition. For these horses, more concentrated sources of energy must be fed. Concentrates containing high levels (5–10 percent) of fat are recommended. Dietary fat provides large amounts of non-sugar calories that performance horses can use readily.

The other two dietary considerations that should be addressed in performance horses are water and electrolyte consumption. Without proper hydration, exercise tolerance plummets. Water should be offered free-choice to performance horses. The possible exception would be immediately after exercise if the horse is extremely hot and wants to gulp water. In this situation, small amounts of water should be given as the horse cools.

Electrolytes are electrically charged particles that run the nervous system of the horse. The primary electrolytes are sodium, chloride, potassium, magnesium, and calcium. They are critical for proper fluid balance, nerve conduction, and muscle contraction. Electrolytes are lost from the body in sweat. The more a horse sweats, the more electrolytes released from the body. If electrolytes are not replaced, horses become fatigued and intolerant to exercise. Electrolytes should be provided to well-hydrated horses prior to exercise. Once the horse has consumed forage and water after exercise, a second dose of electrolytes can be administered.

Summary

Feeding Miniature horses varies little from feeding their large-scale relatives. The principles of feeding are the same, but the portions must be decreased to account for the Miniature's small size. If a nutrition-related question arises, horse owners should seek the advice of a veterinarian well versed in feeds and feeding or an equine nutritionist. Private consultation firms such as Performance Horse Nutrition and Kentucky Equine Research and extension personnel and professors at universities may also offer sound, scientifically-based advice (see Appendix D).

Dwarfism

What is Dwarfism?

BY DEFINITION, A dwarf is any individual, whether human, animal, or plant, that is below the usual accepted size of its species or kind. However, with respect to Miniature horses, a dwarf is not only smaller than normal, it also has varying degrees and combinations of undesirable conformational faults (fig. 9.1). Characteristics of dwarfism in Miniature horses include:

- Lack of lengthening of the legs and neck as the body and head continue to grow. This results in an animal that appears to have an oversized head and body for its height.
- Angular limb and flexural deformities (see *Abnormalities of Growth,* p. 15). These deformities are often severe enough that the horse develops premature arthritis and progressive lameness.
- Abnormal dentition, most commonly sow mouth where the lower jaw protrudes beyond the upper jaw (see *Malocclusions,* p. 53).
- Facial deformities including bulging forehead, extreme facial dish, turned-up nose, nostrils set too high or close together, and overly large and protruding eyes.
- Potbellies with girth depth greater than leg length.
- Enlarged genitals.
- Vertebral deviations including scoliosis (curvature of the spine), kyphosis (roach back), and lordosis (sway back).
- "Low rider" conformation behind, with the height at the withers markedly greater than the height at the croup, which may be severe enough so that the horse is unable to stand on the rear limbs.
- Behavioral abnormalities including inactivity and depression that develop secondary to chronic musculoskeletal pain.

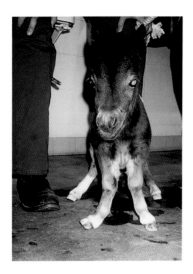

9.1 A dwarf Miniature horse foal. Note the large head in relationship to the body size, angular limb deformities, and flexural deformities. (Photo courtesy of Joanne Kramer, DVM).

A dwarf Miniature horse may have one or a combination of these traits with varying degrees of severity. Mildly affected individuals can lead normal lives, whereas the most severely affected must be euthanized because of chronic pain or the inability to stand or move. In some instances, the deformities are not noticeable at birth, but become obvious as the horse ages.

Care of Dwarf Miniature Horses

There is little question that extremely deformed dwarf foals should be euthanized at birth because they will have difficulty ambulating and will experience a life of chronic pain. However, with proper care, less severely affected individuals can live long, healthy lives and frequently make excellent pets. Angular limb and flexural deformities should be corrected as much as possible (see *Abnormalities of Growth*, p. 15) and proper hoof trimming is essential to minimize stress on the deformed limbs. Many of these horses require the use of acrylic hoof extensions for life to support soft-tissue laxities (see fig. 1.16). Individuals with facial deformities or malocclusions will need frequent dental care to prevent abnormal wear of the teeth and formation of hooks that frequently occur as a result of malocclusions (see *Malocclusions*, p. 53).

Horses with leg or back deformities should not be expected to perform any type of even mildly strenuous work as crippling arthritis can develop quickly in these animals. Similarly, Miniature horses with facial deformities that cause any type of respiratory noise or difficulty breathing should not be asked to exert themselves, especially in hot weather. In general, dwarf Miniature horses or Miniature horses with dwarf characteristics are best suited to be companion animals, not athletic performers.

Genetics

While dwarfism is considered an inherited trait, the exact mode of inheritance has yet to be determined. Because dwarf Miniature horses are frequently a result of the mating of two apparently normal individuals, the presence of a recessive "dwarf gene" has been hypothesized. Not only does this explain a dwarf offspring from normal parents, it also explains how many of these matings have produced completely normal foals before the breeding that resulted in a dwarf foal.

Another possibility is that dwarfism is a result of the interaction of multiple genes. This would explain the different degrees of dwarfism and

how an otherwise normal Miniature horse could have a single dwarf characteristic.

While it is unlikely that any breeder of Miniature horses would argue that a dwarf should not in any circumstances reproduce, how to handle horses with dwarf characteristics, and normal horses that have produced a dwarf, is a bit more complicated. Because of the possibility that horses with dwarf characteristics may be carrying a gene or genes related to dwarfism, they should not enter the breeding pool. For this reason, the AMHA does not accept for registration any horse that exhibits two dwarf characteristics, no matter how mild, or a horse that demonstrates a single severe characteristic.

Ideally, the same should hold true for mares and stallions that produce dwarf foals. However, in reality, dwarfism is an expected by-product of any breeding program whose goal is maintain miniature versions of large animals. Therefore, eliminating all breeding stock that have produced or are related to dwarfs would eradicate a very large portion of the breeding population. Therefore, a reasonable approach would be to not repeat a breeding that has produced a dwarf. In fact, the **dam** of the dwarf should be bred to a stallion that has a totally unrelated bloodline to the **sire** of the dwarf.

Summary

Dwarfism is an unfortunate complication of breeding for miniaturized horses. While severely affected animals are most kindly euthanized, many dwarfs can lead long, healthy lives as companion animals. The likelihood of a breeder producing a dwarf can be reduced by never breeding a dwarf animal or any animal that exhibits any dwarf characteristics. In addition, the mating of a mare and stallion that produced a dwarf should not be repeated.

Normal Physical Parameters

THE FOLLOWING ARE normal parameters for Miniature horses at rest in moderate ambient temperature.

Adult Horses

Heart rate: 34–44 beats per minute; increases in response to exercise or excitement

Respiratory rate: 10–18 breaths per minute; increases in response to exercise or excitement.

Temperature: 99–101 ° F (37.2–38.3 ° C); increases in response to exercise or high environmental temperatures.

Water consumption: 5% of body weight per day; increases in response to exercise and dry or hot weather:

One gallon of water weighs about 8.36 pounds.
One liter of water weighs about 1 kilogram.

Sample calculation for a 175-lb (79.5-kg) Miniature horse.
5% of 175 lbs = 8.75 lbs
8.75 lbs = minimum daily water intake of a little over 1 gallon
5% of 79.5 kg = 4 kg
4 kg = minimum daily water intake of 4 liters

Neonatal Foals

Heart rate: 80–120 beats per minute
Respiratory rate: 30–40 breaths per minute
Temperature: 99–101.8 ° F (37.2–38.8 ° C)
Nursing frequency: every 1–2 hours
Weight gain: about 0.5 lb (1 kg) per day

Poisonous Plants

THE FOLLOWING IS a list of plants where all or part of the plant is toxic to horses.

The toxic effects range from symptoms as mild as excess salivation to those as serious as death. Recognition of poisonous plants is especially important in Miniature horses where, because of their small size, ingestion of even a small amount of toxin can be deadly. Also, Miniature horses are more likely to have access to their owner's yards and gardens where these plants are common.

There may be toxic plants that are not included in this list. Horse owners should contact their local extension agent or veterinarian if they have a question on the safety of particular plants. There are many excellent texts written on toxic plants that include descriptions and photos of plants. More information can also be found on the Cornell University's poisonous plants web pages (www.ansci.cornell.edu/plants/alphalist.html).

The best approach is to remove all weeds from pastures and paddocks and to not allow Miniature horses access to backyards and gardens.

Aconite
Amaryllis Bulbs
Angel's Trumpet
Apple of Peru
Apricot Pits
Arrowgrass
Arum Lily
Azalea
Baneberry
Bird of Paradise Seed Pods
Birdsfoot Trefoil
Black Locust
Black Walnut (*Including Black Walnut shavings*)

Bleeding Heart Foliage and Roots
Bloodroot
Blue Morning Glory
Bouncing Bet
Bracken Fern
Broccoli
Buckeye
Buckwheat
Buffalo Bur
Bull Nettle
Buttercups
Cabbage
Caladium
Candelabra Cactus

Cardinal Flower

Castor Bean Plant

Celandine

Ceriman

Chinaberry Tree

Chives

Cherry (*Choke, Wild, Black, Bitter,*
  and Pin)

Climbing Lily

Climbing Nightshade

Clover (*Alsike, Red, White*)

Christmas Rose

Cocklebur

Corn Cockle

Corn Lily

Cowbane

Cow Cockle

Cowslip

Creeping Charlie

Crown Vetch

Crowfoot

Daffodil Bulbs

Daphne

Death Angel Mushrooms

Death Cap

Death Camas

Delphiniums

Devil's Trumpet

Destroying Angels

Dieffenbachia

Dock

Dogbane

Dolls Eyes

Drooping Leucothoe

Dutchman's Breeches

Eastern Skunk Cabbage

Elderberries

Elephant Ears

English Ivy Berries and Leaves

English Walnut Hulls

Ergot

European Bittersweet

European Mistletoe Berries

False Hellbore

Fiddleneck

Flax

Fly Agaric

Foxglove Leaves

Gill Over The Ground

Golden Chain Bean Capsule

Ground Ivy

Groundsels

Halogeton

Henbane

Horsebrush

Horse Chestnut

Horse Nettle

Horsetail

Hydrangea

Indian Tobacco

Irises

Jack In The Pulpit

Japanese Pieris

Japanese Yew Berries

Jerusalem Cherry Berries

Jessamine Berries

Jimsonweed

Johnson Grass

Klamath Weed

Laburnum

Lamb's Quarters

Lantana Berries

Larkspur

Laurels

Lily Of The Valley

Locoweed

Lobelia

Lucerne

Lupine

Mandrake

Malanga

Marsh Marigold

Marijuana
Mayapple
Milk Bush
Milkweed
Milo
Mistletoe
Monkshood Fleshy Roots
Monkey Agaric
Moonseed Mushrooms *(Amanita spp)*
Mountain Fetterbrush
Mustard
Narcissus Bulbs
Nettlespurge
Nightshade *(Common, Black,
    Belladonna, or Deadly)*
Oak Trees
Oleander
Onions *(Commercial, Wild, Swamp)*
Panther
Panther Cap
Pea *(Sweet, Everlasting, Caley, Tangier,
    and Singletary)*
Peyote
Precatory Bean
Philodendron
Pigweed
Poiseana
Poison Oak, Ivy, and Sumac
Poinsettia Leaves and Stems
Poison Hemlock
Pokeweed
Ponderosa Pine
Poppy *(Prickly, Opium, or Mexican)*
Potato
Privet
Pyracantha
Ragworts
Rape
Red Sage
Red Maple
Rosary Pea

Rhododendron
Rhubarb Leaves
Senecio
Sensitive Fern
Sierra Laurel
Skunk Cabbage
Snakeberry
Snow Drops
Snow-On-The-Mountain
Sorghum
Spurges
Squirrel Corn
Star of Bethlehem
Stinging Nettle
St. John's Wort
Star-Of-Bethlehem
Sudan Grass
Sweet Cherry Seeds
Sweet Clover *(White and Yellow)*
Tall Fescue *(Endophyte infected)*
Tansey Ragwort
Thornapple
Threadleaf Groundsel
Tinsel Tree
Toadstool *(Amanita spp)*
Tobacco
Tree Tobacco
Trumpet Vine
Tung Oil Tree
Turnips
Vetch *(Common, Hairy, Narrow-leaved,
    Purple, and Broad Beans)*
Water Hemlock
White Cohosh
White Snakeroot
Wisteria Seed Pods
Wolfsbane
Yellow Sage
Yellow Star Thistle
Yew Berries and Foliage

Clinical Signs of Disease

THIS TABLE LISTS common symptoms of disease and possible causes in Miniature horses. It is designed to be a quick reference to those diseases and abnormalities discussed in this text. Therefore, it is not an all-inclusive list of possible diseases, but focuses on those of special concern to Miniature horses.

SYMPTOM OF DISEASE	POSSIBLE CAUSES
DEPRESSION AND/OR WEAKNESS	Colic (Ch. 4) Respiratory infection (Ch. 2) Hepatic lipidosis (Ch. 5) Hypothyroidism (Ch. 6) Cushing's disease (Ch. 6) Hypocalcemia (Ch. 7)
FEVER	Infection Colitis (Ch. 4) Hepatic lipidosis (Ch. 5)
LOSS OF APPETITE	Colic (Ch. 4) Respiratory infection (Ch. 2) Hepatic lipidosis (Ch. 5) Tooth root abscess (Ch. 3) Impacted tooth (Ch. 3)
DIARRHEA	Colitis (Ch. 4) Sand impaction (Ch. 4) Enterolith (Ch. 4) Hepatic lipidosis (Ch. 5)

WEIGHT LOSS	Sand colitis (Ch. 4)
	Hepatic lipidosis (Ch. 5)
	Cushing's disease (Ch. 6)
	Hyperthyroidism (Ch. 6)
	Tooth root abscess (Ch. 3)

NASAL DISCHARGE	Respiratory infection (Ch. 2)
	Sinusitis (Ch. 2)
	Tooth root abscess (Ch. 3)

DIFFICULT OR NOISY BREATHING	Respiratory infection (Ch. 2)
	Choanal atresia (Ch. 2)
	Collapsing trachea (Ch. 2)
	Cleft palate (Ch. 2)
	Eruption bumps (Ch. 3)

FACIAL SWELLING	Eruption bumps (Ch. 3)
	Tooth root abscess (Ch. 3)
	Impacted tooth (Ch. 3)
	Sinusitis (Ch. 2)

Resources for Miniature Horse Owners

American Miniature Horse Association
5601 South Interstate 35W
Alvarado, TX 76009
Phone: 817-783-5600
Website: www.minihorses.com/amha/
Email: information@amha.org

American Miniature Horse Registry
81B East Queenwood
Morton, IL 61550
Phone: 309-263-4044
Website: www.shetlandminiature.com/amhr.htm
Email: info@shetlandminiature.com

International Falabella Miniature Horse Society
Holding Hook,
Hampshire RG27 England
Phone: 01256-763425
Website: www.falabella.co.uk/ifmhs.html
Email: ifmhs@falabella.co.uk

Miniature Horse Association of Australia, Inc.
PO Box 3030
Success, 6164 Western Australia
Phone: 61 08 9417 7727
Website:www.geocities.com/qldmhaa/
   Home.html

Miniature Horse Association of Canada
c/o Mary Jo Chapman
RR 1
Holstein, ON N0G 2AO Canada
Phone: 519-334-4007
Website: www.clrc.on.ca/mini.html

The Farrier and Hoofcare Resource Center
1265 Ash Lane
Lebanon, PA 17042
Phone: 717-279-6666
Website: www.horseshoes.com
Email: horseshoes@horseshoes.com

Nanric, Inc.
PO Box 602
Versailles, KY 40383
Phone: 877-462-6742
Website: www.nanric.com
Email: reddenequinefootdoc@att.net

Northern Virginia Equine
Stephen E. O'Grady, DVM, MRCVS
7135 Mt. Eccentric Road
The Plains, VA 20198
Phone: 540-253-5144
Website: www.equipodiatry.com
Email: sogrady@equipodiatry.com

GENERAL INFORMATION ON
MINIATURE HORSES
Miniature Horse World Magazine
Published by American Miniature Horse
Association (see Breed Registries)

Small Horse Press
PO Box 8016
Zanesville, OH 43702
Phone: 800-3759378
Website: www.smallhorse.com
Email: blel@SmallHorse.com

NUTRITION INFORMATION
Kentucky Equine Research, Inc.
3910 Delaney Ferry Road
Versailles, KY 40383
Phone: 800-772-1988
Website: www.ker.com
Email: info@ker.com

Performance Horse Nutrition, LLC
Stephen E. Duren, PhD
967 Haas Road
Weiser, ID 83672
Phone: 208-549-2323
Email: phn@webtrak.com

REPRODUCTION INFORMATION AND
SUPPLIES
Animal Health Care Products
(Predict-A-Foal)
2660 E. 37th Street
Vernon, CA 90058
Phone: 213-583-8981

Classic Medical Supply, Inc.
(Probe handle extension)
19900 Mono Road
Suite 105
Tequesta, FL 33469
Phone: 561-746-9527
Website: www.classicmedical.com
Email: info@classicmed.com

Electronic Animal Management, Inc.
(Birth Alert)
3877 Simonds Road
Corfu, NY 14036
Phone: 800-430-5718
Website: www.eamproducts.com
Email: lesateam@iinc.com

FA Ranch and Racing
(Miniature Artificial Vagina)
5600 Meacham
Carson City, NV 89704
Phone: 775-887-7417

foalert, Inc.
PO Box 2400
Acworth, GA 30102
Website: www.foalert.com
Email: foalert@mindspring.com

Fort Dodge Animal Health
(Pneumabort-K +1b vaccine)
9401 Indian Creek Parkway
Suite 1500
Overland Park, KS 66210
Website:www.wyeth.com/divisions/
   fort_dodge.asp

Intervet Inc. *(Prodigy vaccine)*
405 State Street
Millsboro, DE 19966
Phone: 800-992-8051

Sue McDonnell, PhD
Equine Behavior Lab
University of Pennsylvania School
   of Veterinary Medicine
New Bolton Center
382 West Street Road
Kennett Square, PA 19382
Phone: 610-444-5800
Website:www2.vet.upenn.edu/labs/equine
   behavior/
Email: suemcd@vet.upenn.edu

acute: disease or condition of short duration or recent onset.

acquired: not present at birth, but develops over time.

adhesions: scar tissue that connects two or more anatomic structures such as between two sections of intestine or between a tendon and tendon sheath.

angular limb deformities (ALDs): conformation abnormality that is visible when standing in front of or behind the horse; affects the lower joints of the body so that the limb below the affected joint deviates medially or laterally to the limb above the affected joint.

anorexia: loss of appetite; off feed.

arcade: pertaining to an arch; in dentistry, refers to the collection of teeth in the upper or lower jaw.

bilateral: pertaining to or affecting two sides or both sides.

brachygnathia: overbite; parrot mouth.

bursa: a fluid filled sac that lies over an area of friction, such as between a bone and tendon (example: navicular bursa).

cap: remnant of a deciduous (temporary) tooth that sits on the chewing surface of an erupting permanent tooth.

carpus (*pl carpi*)**:** joint of the forelimb that lays between the radius and cannon bone; equine equivalent of the human wrist.

chronic: disease or condition of long duration, frequently with a slow onset.

club foot: an acquired or congenital con-formational abnormality of the hoof where the angle of the foot is overly upright and the heels are excessively long.

colic: term used to describe abdominal pain; while primarily associated with gastrointestinal disease, may also be caused by abnormalities of the reproductive or urinary systems.

colitis: inflammation of the large intestine.

colostrum: mare's first milk; contains the antibodies that will protect the foal from infection during its first few months of life.

congenital: present at birth

contracture: flexural deformity where the joints of the lower limb are not able to reach full extension due to excessive tension of the flexor tendons and/or suspensory ligament.

cryptorchid: a male animal whose testicle has not descended into its normal position in the scrotum; may be one or both testicles.

cuboidal bones: small, box-shaped bones that make up the carpal and hock joints.

Cushing's disease: disease caused by over-activity of the pituitary gland due to the presence of a benign tumor on that gland.

dam: the female parent of an offspring

deciduous: temporary; in dentistry, used to describe the first set of teeth.

desmotomy: surgical procedure where a ligament is cut.

dwarf: any human, animal, or plant that is below the usual accepted size for its species or kind. In Miniature horses, dwarfs also exhibit undesirable conformation deformities including angular limb deformities, head deformities, and overly short legs.

dystocia: difficult birthing.

endoscope: instrument used to visualize internal structures of the body.

enterolith: concretion of minerals that form in the intestine, usually forms around a foreign body inside the bowel.

erupt: process of a tooth pushing through the gum line into the mouth; cutting a tooth.

eruption bumps: swellings that develop on the jaw or head of a young horse in response to the increased pressure on the skull by the developing permanent teeth.

estrus: period of time in a mare's reproductive cycle where she is receptive to the stallion; fertile period.

fecalith: a firm, fecal-ball-shaped impaction of the small colon.

fetotomy: the process of removing the appendages from a dead foal to extract it from a mare's uterus; used when the foal will not fit through the birth canal because it is over sized or deformed.

fibula: one of the two bones of the rear limb that originate at the stifle; normally fuses with the tibia near the midpoint of the tibia.

float: filing of teeth to remove sharp edges or areas of uneven wear.

flexural deformities: conformational abnormalities that are visible when looking from the side of the horse; may be laxities or contractures.

founder: a complication of laminitis where there is a shifting of the coffin bone away from the hoof wall (rotation or sinking) secondary to inflammation of the soft tissues that attach the coffin bone to the hoof wall.

gestation: time period from conception to delivery of the foal.

gravel: abscess within the soft tissue of the hoof wall; breaks open and drains at the coronary band.

hepatic lipidosis: liver disease caused by excess deposition of fat in the liver cells.

hook: sharp tooth edge that protrudes beyond the border of the opposing tooth; caused by uneven tooth wear.

hormone: a chemical substance that is produced and secreted by one organ then transported in the blood stream to another organ or body part, thereby affecting the function or activity of that organ or body part.

hyperlipemia: a disease characterized by increased levels of fat products (triglycerides, cholesterol, fatty acids) in the blood.

hyper: prefix indicating increased or excessive.

hypo: prefix indicating decreased or insufficient .

hypoplasia: incomplete formation or development.

impacted: tightly lodged in place; can be used to describe a tooth that cannot erupt due to compression by adjacent teeth or blockage of the gastrointestinal tract preventing normal movement of fecal material.

impedance: resistance to flow.

inguinal canal: slit in the abdominal wall located in the groin area at the top of the thigh (one on each side); testicle passes from the abdomen through this slit during fetal development.

internal fixation: surgical procedure where metal devices (plates, screws, pins) are placed under the skin to stabilize fractures.

laminitis: inflammation of the soft tissue of the foot that connects the coffin bone to the hoof wall; severe cases result in rotation or sinking of the coffin bone away from the hoof wall (founder).

lateral: anatomical descriptor of position indicating an area away from the middle of the body (example: the outside of a horse's leg is the lateral side).

laxity: flexural deformity caused by lack of support from the flexor tendons and/or suspensory ligament.

ligament: connective tissue band that runs from bone to bone.

luxation: dislocation.

malocclusion: dental abnormality where the teeth do not align evenly.

meconium: a foal's first feces; produced while the foal is developing in the uterus and consists of sloughed intestinal cells, mucous, and bile.

medial: anatomical descriptor of position indicating an area closer to the middle of the body (example: the inside of the leg is the medial side).

neonate: newborn animal that is less than 28 days of age.

nonsteroidal anti-inflammatory drugs (NSAIDs): a group of medications that act to decrease fever, relieve pain, and decrease inflammation (examples: aspirin, phenylbutazone, flunixin meglumine).

occlusal: the surface of a tooth that contacts the opposing arcade; chewing surface.

ossification: formation of bone from a cartilage or fibrous tissue precursor.

palpation: to examine using the hands and fingers; to feel.

parrot mouth: dental malocclusion where the upper incisors protrude in front of the lower incisors; overbite.

parturition: the birthing process; labor.

periarticular: surrounding the joint; used to describe soft tissue structures that surround the joint including ligaments and the joint capsule.

periosteum: soft tissue covering of bone, provides blood supply to the surface of the bone and has bone-forming activity in growing animals.

physis (pl physes): growth plate

physeal: of or relating to the physis.

prognathia: underbite; sow mouth.

prosthesis: an artificial substitute for an anatomic structure or part.

quittor: draining tract near the heel or quarter of the foot, caused by an infected collateral cartilage.

radius (pl. radii): long bone of the forearm.

radiograph: an image produced by the action of X rays on a specialized film.

repulsion: extraction of a tooth by creating a hole in the skull above the root and hammering the tooth out of the skull.

serum: fluid portion of the blood that remains after removal of the clotting factors and cellular components.

sinusitis: sinus infection

sire: the male parent of an offspring.

sow mouth: dental malocclusion where the lower incisors protrude in front of the upper incisors; underbite.

systemic: of or relating to the whole body; when used to describe a medication protocol, it means that the medication is delivered to the whole body as opposed to local application.

tendon: a connective tissue band that runs from muscle to bone.

tendon sheath: fluid filled soft tissue envelope surrounding a tendon; usually located where a tendon passes over a bony prominence or joint; secretes a thick, slippery fluid that creates a slick surface for the free movement of the tendon.

transverse ridges: enamel corrugations that run in a regular, repeating pattern on the chewing surface of a horse's cheek teeth.

ulna: one of the two bones of the forearm; normally fuses with the radius near the midpoint of the radius.

unilateral: of or pertaining to one side.

INDEX

ABOUT THE AUTHOR

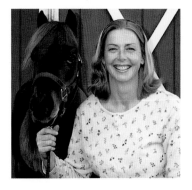

DR. REBECCA FRANKENY has spent her entire adult life working with horses. After twelve years as an exercise rider, groom, assistant trainer, and eventually a trainer of Thoroughbred racehorses, she entered veterinary school at the University of Pennsylvania. It was during her years as a veterinary student that she was first introduced to Miniature horses and their unique medical concerns. Since then she has had 10 years of clinical experience working with Miniature horses, including a three-year equine surgery residency at the University of Missouri. Her fondness and appreciation for the breed became firmly established after becoming a Miniature horse owner.

Dr. Frankeny is currently the surgeon at Comstock Large Animal Hospital. In addition to her clinical duties, she also writes the hospital's bi-annual newsletter and organizes client continuing education. She is an adjunct faculty member at the University of Nevada, Reno where she teaches equine medicine to pre-veterinary students and animal science majors. She is a frequent guest speaker at equine association meetings throughout Nevada.

Dr. Frankeny lives in Reno, Nevada with her husband Mike, their cat, three dogs, and two horses.